EMS

ESSENTIALS

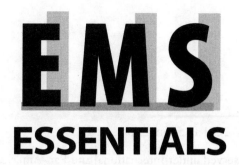

EMS
ESSENTIALS

A Portable Glossary

Debra Cason

New York

Library of Congress Cataloging-in-Publication Data:
Cason, Debra.
    EMS essentials : a portable glossary / Debra Cason with Mary Masi.
        p. cm.
    ISBN 1-57685-385-3 (pbk.)
    1. Emergency medical technicians—Examinations—Study guides. 2. Emergency medicine—Dictionaries.   I. Masi, Mary. II. Title.
RA645.5 .C376 2001
616.02'5'076—dc21   2001033885

Printed in the United States of America
9 8 7 6 5 4 3 2 1
First Edition

For more information or to place an order, contact LearningExpress at:
    900 Broadway
    Suite 604
    New York, NY 10003

Or visit us at:
    www.learnatest.com

About the Authors

Debra Cason is Past President of the National Association of Emergency Medical Service Educators (NAEMSE). Ms. Cason is currently Associate Professor, Health Care Sciences and Program Director, Emergency Medicine Education at the University of Texas Southwestern Medical Center at Dallas. She is a Registered Nurse, EMT-Paramedic, and an EMT-Paramedic Course Coordinator-Texas. Over her distinguished career, Ms. Cason has enjoyed numerous professional appointments and has graced many national education and accreditation commissions as Chair, Commissioner, and Board member. Ms. Cason has also published extensively on training and education issues specific to EMS.

Mary Masi is the founder of InfoSurge, a company specializing in writing, research, and editorial consulting. Previously, she worked in the editorial division of John Wiley & Sons, and as a college writing instructor. Ms. Masi has also authored several LearningExpress titles, including the *Firefighter Career Starter*.

Contents

Chapter 1 How to Use This Book to Get a Top Score   1

Chapter 2 Studying for Success   11

Chapter 3 Mnemonics   41

Chapter 4 EMS Glossary   61

Appendix Axial Skeleton   113

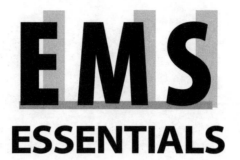

ESSENTIALS

chapter **1**

How to Use This Book to Get a Top Score

Are you thinking about how to get ready for an upcoming emergency medical service (EMS) exam? Do you need some help in putting all the pieces of test preparation together? If so, this book will give you the EMS knowledge that you need, whether you are new to the field or have been an experienced EMS professional for many years.

Perhaps you want to become certified as a first responder and you've never had any medical training. You can use this book as a study guide and methodically work your way through it from cover to cover, learning about a range of topics, from finding out new study strategies and memory tricks to using the terms in the glossary to create flash cards and study lists.

On the other hand, you may already have many years of experience as an emergency medical technician (EMT)-Basic or EMT-Intermediate, but you want to gain the advanced certification of an EMT-Paramedic. If that's the case, you can use this book to brush up on basic study skills and to pick up some new ideas for different ways to remember medical terminology. You can use the glossary as a reference as needed during your review of EMS materials.

Or you may be somewhere between these two extremes. Either way, this book offers you a wealth of EMS information, and it is likely that you will return to it as a reference and guide for many years to come.

YOUR UPCOMING EMS EXAM

Let's take a closer look at the written EMS exam(s) that you may need to take to enter or further your EMS career. A written exam is a certification requirement for becoming an EMS provider at one of the following four levels:

1. First Responder
2. EMT-Basic
3. EMT-Intermediate
4. EMT-Paramedic

The National Registry of Emergency Medical Technicians (NREMT) sets uniform national standards for training, testing, and continuing education for EMS professionals at each of these four levels. The NREMT is a not-for-profit, nongovernmental, free-standing agency led by a board of directors. Some directors are members of national EMS organizations, whereas others have expertise in EMS systems.

The NREMT began in 1970 and has examined over 750,000 EMTs since its inception. You can become registered with the NREMT by meeting the current entry requirements, which include passing written and performance examinations. There are about 155,000 EMS providers who are currently registered with the NREMT. Registration continues if you complete education and experience requirements and forward necessary applications on a biannual basis. You can visit the NREMT website for more information, www.nremt.org.

All states test individuals seeking to become EMS providers. Some states make sole use of NREMT tests, while others offer state tests. However, in all 50 states, the NREMT works together with states' offices of Emergency Medical Services to establish certification requirements for EMS providers.

The curriculum for EMS education and testing comes from the Department of Transportation National Highway Traffic Safety Administration National Standard Curriculum.

All four written tests used by the National Registry to examine prospective EMS professionals are in a multiple-choice question format. For each exam, you must get an overall score of 70 percent to pass. Table 1.1 gives a breakdown of the topics and number of multiple-choice questions in each topic for the NREMT's EMS written exams:

Contact the NREMT to get an application and to find out where you can take the exam in your state for the level of certification you want. You can also check in career guides, such as the *EMT Career Starter*, 2nd Edition (LearningExpress, New York, 2001) for more information about certification and schooling. Some websites, such as LearnATest.com or emsvillage.com also have information about certification and testing. In addition, the NREMT will tell you how to arrange to take the appropriate EMS examination. In many cases, you

TABLE 1.1   NREMT Written Exams

First-Responder Exam	Number of Questions
Patient Assessment	16–20
Airway and Breathing	16–20
Circulation	15–19
Musculoskeletal, Behavioral, Neurological, and Environmental	14–18
Children and Childbirth	13–17
EMS Systems, Ethical, Legal, Communications, Documentation, Safety, and Triage/Transportation	14–18
TOTAL QUESTIONS	**100**

EMT-Basic Exam	Number of Questions
Airway and Breathing	25–31
Cardiology	24–30
Trauma	23–29
Medical	21–27
Obstetrics and Pediatrics	18–24
Operations	21–27
TOTAL QUESTIONS	**150**

EMT-Intermediate Exam	Number of Questions
Airway and Breathing	24–30
Cardiology	24–30
Trauma	21–29
Medical	21–27
Obstetrics and Pediatrics	19–25
Operations	21–27
TOTAL QUESTIONS	**150**

EMT-Paramedic Exam	Number of Questions
Airway and Breathing	27–33
Cardiology	30–36
Trauma	26–34
Medical	26–34
Obstetrics and Pediatrics	24–32
Operations	26–32
TOTAL QUESTIONS	**180**

will be referred to your state's EMS office, but in other cases you will be instructed to make individual arrangements to take your exam.

National Registry of Emergency Medical Technicians, Inc.
Rocco V. Morando Building
P. O. Box 29233
Columbus, OH 43229
614-888-4484
www.nremt.org

HOW THIS BOOK CAN HELP YOU

The entire process of preparing for an EMS exam, which can seem overwhelming at first glance, can actually be broken down into several manageable steps. This book guides you through each of those steps. The first step is to finish orienting yourself with this introductory chapter. Then, move on to Chapter 2, which explains how to set up an individualized study plan and presents specific study strategies you can use during each study session. You'll learn the steps to take to maximize your chances for scoring high on your upcoming exam. You'll find out when to take sample tests so you can check your scores and still have enough time to focus on the areas in which you need more work. You'll also increase your understanding and retention of the EMS material you are studying by using many different study strategies, not just one or two.

While you are reading Chapter 2, take the time to create an individualized study plan that will fit your needs and schedule. This is a crucial step in the test preparation process. Also, be sure to take at least one practice exam from an EMS test-preparation book, as recommended in the sample study plan. After you finish reading Chapter 2, spend some time using each different study strategy explained in that chapter.

Chapter 3 will show you how to create, use, organize, and review mnemonic devices, which are memory tricks that can help you to overcome memory blocks during an EMS exam. Mnemonics such as acronyms and acrostics can help you score extra points by helping you remember lists and terms when you need to. As you'll find out from Chapter 3, mnemonics are best used *after* you've become familiar with specific EMS material; they should not be used to learn brand new material.

After you finish reading Chapter 3, it's time to tackle the glossary section, which makes up the bulk of this book. The glossary contains a wealth of essential EMS terms that you'll be either learning for the first time or reviewing. If you are new to the EMS field, this glossary of terms may become the backbone of your study sessions. You'll need to learn, or at least become familiar with, most of the terms in this section of the book. If you are an experienced EMS provider who is seeking intermediate or advanced certification, this portion of the book will be a valuable reference and review tool during your study sessions.

USE THIS BOOK WITH OTHER TEST PREPARATION MATERIAL

This book is best used in conjunction with other test preparation material. *EMS Essentials* fills an important gap left by many test-preparation books that do not contain glossaries of terms. Additionally, most test-preparation books do not explain specific study strategies or show how mnemonic devices can help you remember difficult medical terminology.

That said, if you are committed to becoming an EMS worker, you should also invest the time and money into buying and using a test-preparation book that includes several practice EMS exams so that you get the best of both types of study material. Put them together, and you have a winning combination that can help you get a top score on your exam. See Chapter 2 for specific guidance on how to fit practice exams into your study schedule. You'll find a variety of test-preparation books at your local bookstore or library, or you can order them online. Here are suggested titles of test-preparation books:

First Responder
Bergeron, J. D. and Bizjak, G. (2000). *First Responder*, (6th ed.) Upper Saddle River, NJ: Prentice Hall. Book with CD-ROM for Windows & Macintosh.

EMT-Basic
The Complete Preparation Guide to the EMT-Basic Exam (2nd ed.) (2001). New York: LearningExpress.

EMT-Intermediate
Westfal, R.E. (Ed.). (1998). *EMT-Intermediate: Pretest, Self-Assessment and Review* New York: McGraw Hill.

EMT-Paramedic
The Complete Preparation Guide to the Paramedic Exam (2nd ed.) (2001). New York: LearningExpress.

In addition, the Internet also contains a wealth of test-preparation resources for EMS exams. Some sites even offer online practice exams, complete with answer explanations, personalized scoring, and individual analysis. Many tests are now computer based, meaning that when you go to take the exam you will take it on the computer. Therefore, online practice tests are not only a valuable learning tool, but they can also help you become familiar with and feel prepared for the official test, come test day.

After reading and studying this book and taking several practice EMS exams, you'll be well on your way to getting a top score on your upcoming EMS exam. Good luck as you enter or further your rewarding and worthwhile EMS career!

chapter 2

Studying for Success

D o you want to unlock the secrets of how to study for an EMS exam? If so, you've come to the right place. This chapter explains how to create a study plan and gives you specific strategies you can use to make the most of each study session as you prepare for your upcoming EMS exam.

The first step to successful studying is to set up a study plan. In other words, take a few minutes to create a study schedule for yourself. This will allow you to get an overview of what you need to accomplish and what your deadlines are. If you don't know where you're going, how are you ever going to get there? Therefore, the time you spend developing a study plan will serve you well.

Take a moment to think about your goal. Most likely, your goal is to pass an EMS provider examination, either First Responder, EMT-Basic, EMT-Intermediate, or EMT-Paramedic. So let's work backward from that end result of passing your exam. How much time do you have? Can you plan out a leisurely schedule of study for several months or do you need to buckle down and get some serious studying done in a few weeks or less?

An important aspect of a study plan is flexibility. Your plan should help you, not hinder you, so be prepared to alter your study schedule once you get started on it if needed. You'll probably find that one or more steps will take longer to complete than you had anticipated, whereas others will go more quickly.

CREATING YOUR STUDY PLAN

Take a look at the following sample study plan to help you create your own individualized study schedule. Each step of your plan should be flexible, but you can use this timeline as a guide. If you have more time, you can expand the plan; if you have less time, you can compress it.

Sample Study Plan

This schedule is appropriate if you have approximately four to six months before your EMS examination test date.

Four to Six Months Before the Test

Read Chapters 1 to 3 of this book.

Request all materials needed for your test.

Buy a large calendar and mark the date of your test on it. Highlight or clearly emphasize the date with a bright color pen so it stands out every time you glance at the calendar. You can also use a calendar on your computer.

Purchase or borrow an EMS test-preparation book that will help you to prepare for the examination. Titles of suggested books and online resources are listed in Chapter 1.

Take a practice test either online or from your test-preparation book, and carefully check your score. Note how you performed on the different topics appearing on the test. Create a graph or chart that has ample room to record several test scores. Save this chart so you can log each of your practice test scores on it.

Get in the habit of studying your EMS materials every day. It's better to study 20 minutes every day of the week than to save up all those minutes and cram several hours of study into one day on the weekend.

Experiment with using different study strategies discussed in this chapter. Perhaps you want to try a different one each week. Then, when you find out what works the best for you, use that method for the rest of your studies.

Two to Three Months Before the Test

Set aside a specific amount of time each day to review test areas you need to concentrate on to improve your score. Even if you can only squeeze in 15–20 minutes a day, those minutes add up over the course of a week and can dramatically improve your knowledge. Continue using a variety of study strategies during your study sessions.

Take another practice test either online or from an EMS test-preparation book. Record your score on the graph or chart you created. Are your scores steadily going up or are they uneven? Note which type of questions you got wrong so you can review those areas.

Try to enlist the help of a friend or relative who will quiz you on important words and concepts you are studying. Your friend can use the glossary in this book to quiz you on a variety of terms and their definitions.

One Month Before the Test

Confirm the date and location of your exam.

Confirm that your application to take the exam has been received and that you have been sent all the necessary materials.

Make sure you know where the test will be held and how you will get to the test site.

Continue to spend at least 15 minutes every day studying and reviewing EMS material. If you can manage to spend more time in review sessions each day, that is even better. However, if you have been reviewing regularly for a couple of months, the reviews should take you less time since you are so familiar with the material. This is the most important part of studying for tests. The more familiar you are with the information that will be on the test, the better you will perform under test conditions.

Seek support and encouragement from those closest to you. If you live with others, remind them that you have a big test coming up and you need quiet time to study.

One Week Before the Test

Take two more practice tests either online or from an EMS test-preparation book. See how your scores compare with the tests you took at the beginning of your study plan. Try not to become anxious if your score is lower than you think it should be at this point. The reality is that you *do* know more than when you started studying, and it will show when you actually take the test.

Concentrate on being well rested and relaxed about taking the test. Avoid stress and anxiety as much as possible. Each time you find yourself worrying about the test, say to yourself, "I am well prepared and I will do well on this test." Remember, you have been studying hard for the past several months, using this book and other EMS test-preparation material; if you have been keeping to your study plan, you should be well-prepared for your test. Thinking positive thoughts each day can help prepare you mentally for doing well on the test.

Continue your daily study sessions. Even if you feel that you already understand all of the material, you can spend time reviewing and creating mnemonics. (You'll learn more about mnemonics in the next chapter.)

Make sure you have all necessary items—pencils, watch, a sweater, and so on—and have arranged for plenty of time to get to the test site.

STUDY STRATEGIES YOU CAN USE

After you develop a study plan, the next step to successful studying is to decide what specific things you want to do during your study sessions. Using a variety of study strategies rather than simply reading and rereading your textbook can help you make the material come alive so that you can thoroughly understand it. You can also avoid boredom during your study sessions by using many different study methods. Perhaps you want to use a different study strategy each time you sit down to study, or you could use a variety of study strategies throughout the day. For example, you could rewrite some notes in the morning, carry flash cards along with you during the day for those times when you find a few free minutes, and create some sample study questions during your evening study session.

Some study strategies will appeal to you more than

Stay Out of the Cram Trap

By creating a study plan, you can avoid the panic of cramming. Trying frantically to learn all the material you need to know the night before your big exam can frazzle your nerves and leave you too exhausted to do your best on test day.

others. However, give each strategy a chance by trying it at least once, because even if it doesn't look appealing at first glance, you might be surprised and end up enjoying it. The rest of this chapter discusses specific study strategies you can use. Each strategy can help you understand and remember the material you need to know to ace your upcoming EMS exam.

Asking Questions

Asking questions is a powerful study strategy because it forces you to get actively involved in the material you want to learn. Getting actively involved will help you to better understand and remember that material when test time comes around. Another benefit of asking questions is that you may end up asking (and then answering) some of the very same questions that will appear on your exam.

Here are five sample questions you can ask yourself while reading and reviewing EMS material:

1. What is the main idea from this section?
2. How does the information in this section relate to other information I already know?
3. What are the key terms in this section that I should memorize?
4. What are the facts from this section that I need to know for the exam?
5. How can I turn these facts into questions?

Of course, not all the questions you ask about the material you are studying will appear on an exam; however, you will find that many of your questions will at least be related to information tested on the exam. It is much better to ask and answer

18

specific questions than to aimlessly read and reread the text
without any goal in mind.

If you're having trouble coming up with questions based
on the material you are studying, get out a test-preparation
book that contains sample EMS exams and read through several
of the questions. The more practice tests you take, the more
familiar you will become with the types of questions you can
form from your material.

To give you an idea of how to create specific questions
regarding material you are reading, take a look at the four sample questions that follow this paragraph about burns:

> There are three different kinds of burns: first degree,
> second degree, and third degree. It is important for
> EMS professionals to be able to recognize each of these
> types of burns so that they can be sure burn victims are
> given proper treatment. The least serious burn is the
> first-degree burn, which causes skin to turn red but
> does not cause blistering. A mild sunburn is a good ex-
> ample of a first-degree burn, and, like a mild sunburn,
> first-degree burns generally do not require medical
> treatment other than a gentle cooling of the burned
> skin with ice or cold tap water. Second-degree burns,
> on the other hand, do cause blistering of the skin and
> should be treated immediately. These burns should be
> immersed in warm water and then wrapped in a sterile
> dressing or bandage. (Do not apply butter or grease to
> these burns; despite the old wives' tale, butter does *not*
> help burns heal and actually increases chances of infec-
> tion.) If second-degree burns cover a large part of the
> body, then the victim should be taken to the hospital
> immediately for medical care. Third-degree burns are
> those that char the skin and turn it black, or burn so

deeply that the skin shows white. These burns usually result from direct contact with flames and have a great chance of becoming infected. All third-degree burns should receive immediate hospital care. They should not be immersed in water, and charred clothing should not be removed from the victim. If possible, a sterile dressing or bandage should be applied to burns before the victim is transported to the hospital.

Sample Questions
1. What would be a good title for this paragraph?
2. What should second-degree burns be treated with?
3. First-degree burns turn the skin what color?
4. What is the main idea of this paragraph?

By asking questions about the material you read, you help cement into your mind the facts and ideas contained in that material. You can even go a step further and actually come up with multiple-choice questions. Your multiple-choice questions can be adapted from questions you've already asked yourself about the material, or they can cover new topics. Creating multiple-choice questions gives you the chance to step into the role of a teacher (or test developer) and actually practice coming up with a correct answer in the face of several distractors (the other answer choices that are incorrect). Here's an example of the type of multiple-choice questions you could create based on the burn questions asked above:

1. Which of the following would be the best title for this passage?
   a. Dealing with Third-degree Burns
   b. How to Recognize and Treat Different Burns

    c. Burn Categories

    d. Preventing Infection in Burns

2. Second-degree burns should be treated with

    a. butter.

    b. nothing.

    c. cold water.

    d. warm water.

3. First-degree burns turn the skin

    a. red.

    b. blue.

    c. black.

    d. white.

4. Which of the following best expresses the main idea of the paragraph?

    a. There are three different types of burns.

    b. EMS professionals should always have cold compresses on hand.

    c. Different burns require different types of treatment.

    d. Butter is not good for healing burns.

Now comes the fun part: answering the questions! (The answers for the above questions are: 1. **b**, 2. **d**, 3. **a**, 4. **c**.) By the time you've gone through the process of developing questions based on a section of material you want to learn, you will probably already have a good idea of what the answers are. However, it's always a good idea to read through your questions to see if you can answer them without having to look back at the material. You can use your list of questions each time you want to review the material. If time permits, you can also ask additional questions during your review of the material.

You may want to keep all your written questions in a separate place (such as a three-ring binder, folder, or notebook), or include them alongside your notes in a notebook that you use in class or while studying your texts. One format for organizing your questions is to write down your questions and answers on sheets of paper that you can fold in half. Write your questions on the left side and brief answers on the right side. That way, you can fold the paper with the answers underneath to quiz yourself.

After you ask and answer several questions about a topic you are studying, set the questions aside for a few days. Then, without looking at the answers, ask yourself the same questions again and see how many you can answer correctly. Write down additional questions as they come to mind during your review. Often, your search for the answers to your questions will lead to more questions. However, the more questions you ask, the more answers you'll find, and the more material you will know on exam day.

Taking Notes

Taking notes in class or on what you read will help you to understand and remember the information you need to know on exam day. Proper note taking develops your thinking skills. It helps you to listen better, organize material, and recall, digest, and interpret information.

The secret to taking good notes is knowing what is

important enough to write down—and what is not. Three things that are important enough to record are:

1. Main ideas and secondary ideas
2. Authorities
3. Opinions and Facts

When you are sitting in class, listen closely for main points. Learn to separate them from minor, or supporting, points. A good instructor will identify main points for you, but sometimes you have to do this on your own. Here are some verbal clues that point toward a main or important idea:

"The reason is . . ."
"An important factor . . ."
"There are four things to consider . . ."
"The thing to remember . . ."
"The best (or worse, biggest, smallest, last, only, and so on) . . ."

Secondary ideas are often buried in examples, so always be alert to this fact when an instructor offers up an example, especially one that follows something you have identified as a main point.

Other details worth recording in your notes are authorities. Authorities are experts, research studies, and other sources that lend weight to ideas and concepts. It is important not only to write down the ideas or issues that they bring to light, but also to note that this material comes from an authority and/or expert. Take the time to identify the authority in your notes.

You should also listen for and write down in your notes opinions and facts. Facts are bits of information that are real or actual. Mainly they are provable, demonstrable pieces of information. In contrast, opinions are beliefs or conclusions held by someone that may not be objective or proven yet. It may be your opinion that facts are more important than opinions, but this is not necessarily so. An opinion on the future of nuclear physics that emanated from the mouth of the world's most prominent nuclear physicist, for example, would not be something to scoff at. What is important to you as a notetaker is to be sure you identify what is opinion and what is fact. Furthermore, although facts are supposed to be objective, everyone knows there is little truly objective information in this world. Any time you question a fact or an opinion, be sure to put a question mark in your notes, so you can follow up on this point later.

Taking notes is not simply a matter of recording everything you hear. It is a process of absorbing information, assessing it, analyzing it, and then, finally, writing it down so that your notes reflect this process. To do this, begin to outline what you are hearing in your mind as you hear it, and before you write it down.

Depending on the speaking skills of your instructor, you may need to work harder or less hard to understand what he or she has to say and then translate this into useful notes. Here are three strategies that instructors use to organize their lectures. Use the strategies to help you organize your notes.

1. Beginning—middle—end
2. Relevant—irrelevant
3. Theme—subtheme

Most lectures have a beginning, a middle, and an end. This is something you can listen for, and then structure your notes around. Try to divide what you hear, and also what you write down, into these three categories.

Some instructors tend to throw in irrelevant material during their lectures. Much of this does not belong in your notes and is a waste of time to write. Learn to weed out irrelevant material. This is easier said than done because irrelevant material is not always easy to identify. For instance, some instructors use anecdotes to make important points. In these cases, you may have to listen for a few minutes to realize that an instructor is making an important point worth recording. A good strategy for taking notes is to take notes during class in a draft notebook. Then, after class, go through, reorganize, and rewrite your notes into a final-notes notebook.

Other instructors organize their lectures around themes and subthemes. If your instructor is organized, the difference between themes and subthemes will be obvious. If your instructor is disorganized, however, you'll have to write all the themes down and then go back over them after the lecture to identify which points are main themes and which are subthemes.

Mapping Information

A map is a visual way of recording information you hear or read. Indeed, you can map information about anything you are studying, whether you are in a classroom listening to a lecture or you are sitting in the library reading a textbook. If you enjoy visualizing, this is a good study strategy for you because when you draw a map of information, the relationships between topics become clearly visible.

The good news is that you don't have to be an artist to draw an effective map. The process is really quite straightforward. The first step is to get out a clean sheet of paper. Then, in the middle of that piece of paper, write down the main point, idea, or topic under consideration. Draw a circle around this main topic. Next, draw branches out from that center circle on which to record subtopics and details. Create as many branches as you need or as many as will fit on your sheet of paper! Below is an example of a simple map; it has only one level of subheadings.

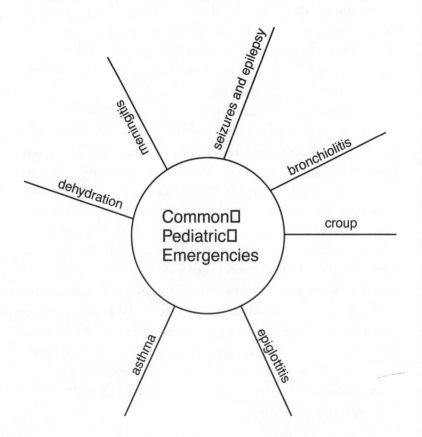

The level of detail you'll include on each map depends on what you want to remember. Perhaps you already know part of a subject thoroughly but can't seem to remember any details about one or two particular subtopics. In that case, you can tailor the map to fit your needs. For example, consider a student who has studied seven common pediatric emergencies. He is very familiar with five of them: bronchiolitis, asthma, seizures and epilepsy, meningitis, and epiglottitis. However, he is having trouble remembering two of them: croup and dehydration. This student may want to draw a map that includes all of the pediatric emergencies. However, the map should also include specific details about the two subtopics that he has trouble recalling. An example of this type of map is opposite.

Mapping information forces you to organize the information you are studying, whether that information is from your class notes, a special EMS lecture, field visit, or an EMS textbook. Sometimes, you'll find that you need to spend considerable time to come up with an appropriate phrase, word, or sentence to write in the center circle of a map. Then you may need to spend even more time considering which topics are related to that main topic for the next level of branches. It is a process of making decisions and connections between ideas and facts. That process alone makes drawing maps an effective study strategy. Another benefit is that after you complete a map, you have an excellent review aid. Because the material on a map is organized in a visual way, you will be able to recall that information more readily each time you review it. It gives the material you are studying a definite structure.

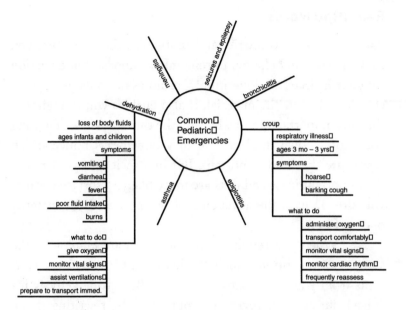

One way to use a map as a review aid is to take one out and study it carefully for five to ten minutes. Then, put it out of sight and attempt to recreate the entire map from memory. By forcing yourself to recall the items on the map, you ensure that those items are learned. You may find additional information to add to the map while you search through your memory for the actual data you saw on the map.

Another way you can use a map you created is to review it several days or weeks later. At that time, add more details to the map. You can look through a textbook or your notes to find additional information about the topic on your map, and pull out additional information to add to the map that you didn't include when you originally created the map.

Rewriting Notes

Taking the time to rewrite and reorganize the notes that you took in class can help you to remember important information for your EMS exam. Rewriting your notes not only gives you a chance to review the material, it also enables you to highlight the most important points. During the time-pressure of getting your notes down in class, you may not always notice which points are the most important. But in a review of your notes, the important ideas and facts are more likely to surface because you already have the advantage of having heard the material once before.

When you rewrite your notes, you are employing the strategy of repetition, which will help you to cement key concepts from your notes into your brain. By getting actively involved during your review of your notes by rewriting them, you log much more information into your memory than if you merely read through your notes.

Another benefit of rewriting your notes is that you can write them more legibly because you will have more time to write in a study session than in class. This is especially helpful if you find that you are rushing in class to get your notes written and can't take the time to write carefully.

One way to rewrite your notes is to take your hand-written notebook pages to a computer to type them up in an organized format. Just follow these eight steps:

1. While you're at the keyboard, take a few moments to think about your notes before you begin to type.

How to SCORE When Rewriting Your Notes!

Select	Select only the important information from your notes when you are in the process of rewriting them. Don't copy your notes verbatim.
Condense	Shorten long paragraphs or lists by writing a brief summary about the material.
Organize	Create headings and subheadings, and rearrange the material in your notes to make it organized.
Rephrase	Use your own words as much as possible—especially if you tend to take notes without rephrasing the instructor's words.
Evaluate	As you rewrite your notes, take time to evaluate their effectiveness. If they seem lacking on a particular topic that was covered in class, ask a classmate if you can see his or her notes too.

2. Come up with a title for the topic or topics your notes cover, and type this at the top of the page.

3. Continue to read through your notes, and each time you see an important point, key that point into the computer. It helps if you change the wording slightly. Paraphrasing your own notes

will help you to better understand and remember the material.

4. Add headings to separate topics.
5. Use **bold** or ALL CAPS to emphasize key points.
6. Change information from straight text into bullet points or numbered lists when possible. This can speed your review when you come back to look at your typed notes.
7. Print out the notes when you are finished and save them in a file, folder, or three-ring binder.
8. Review your typewritten notes regularly.

Creating Flash Cards

Creating flash cards to use as a study aid is a simple yet highly effective way to learn information. You may want to get creative when you sit down to create flash cards. For instance, you can use different-sized cards for different subjects, such as 4x6 for airway and breathing topics and 3x5 cards for pediatric topics. Or, you can use different colored index cards to organize your study material according to topic.

The beauty of creating index cards is that you can carry them with you throughout the day, especially the small cards that will fit into your backpack or purse. You may want to rotate the cards that you carry with you, so you can get through them all without having to carry a thick pile of cards every day. The number of flash cards you create is limited only by your time and inclination. You could conceivably create a flash card for every term in the glossary in this book.

The following are two examples of how to create your own set of flash cards:

Front of Card

The central nervous system consists of

Back of Card

the brain and spinal cord

Front of Card

Signs and symptoms of possible head trauma

Back of Card

seizures confusion irregularly dilated pupils bruising around eyes and ears irregular breathing

Making Outlines

Creating outlines of the material you want to review can help you to organize that material in an orderly way. In addition, outlining gives you another tactic for studying and reviewing your EMS material. The outlining strategy is similar to the rewriting-your-notes strategy. The main difference is that outlines are more formal than notes. That is, there is a certain way outlines should be organized. Organizing information in outline form helps you remember ideas and see the relationships between those ideas. In an outline, you can see exactly how supporting information is related to main ideas.

The basic structure for an outline is this:

I. Topic
  A. Main Idea
    1. Major supporting idea
      a. Minor supporting idea

Outlines can have many layers and many variations, but this is essentially how they work: you start with the topic, move to the main idea, add the major supporting idea, and then list minor supporting ideas (if they seem important enough to write down). When you're working with a larger body of information, the overall main idea (topic) should be at the top. Here's an example of a partially completed outline:

I. Common Pediatric Medical Emergencies
  A. Croup
    1. Respiratory illness occurring in children ages 3 months to 3 years old
    2. Symptoms
      a. hoarse
      b. barking cough
    3. What to do
      a. administer oxygen
      b. transport patient in a comfortable position
      c. monitor vital signs and cardiac rhythm
      d. reassess patient frequently
  B. Dehydration
    1. Loss of body fluids that can occur in both infants and children
    2. Symptoms
      a. vomiting
      b. diarrhea

   c. fever

   d. burns

   e. poor fluid intake

  3. What to do

   a. move patient to shaded area

   b. monitor vital signs

   c. give plenty of fluids

   d. prepare to transport patient immediately

 C. Epiglottitis

  1. Inflammation of the epiglottis that can occur in children ages 3 to 7

  2. Symptoms

   a. appears to be critically ill

   b. sitting upright, leaning forward in a tripod position

   c. mouth is open with a protruding tongue

   d. drooling

   e. respiratory distress or hypoxia

  3. What to do

   a. keep child comfortable and calm

   b. administer oxygen

   c. monitor vital signs and cardiac rhythm

   d. may need to ventilate using positive pressure

 D. Asthma

 E. Bronchiolitis

 F. Seizures and Epilepsy

 G. Meningitis

Outlining a text or your notes enables you to see the different layers of information and how they work together to support the overall main idea. Knowing and remembering the organization of facts can aid you greatly in your test preparation.

Using Highlighters

Another study strategy you can use to review important material for your upcoming exam is to use highlighters and markers to mark up your textbook, test-preparation books, and notes. Marking the material you want to remember can help you to focus on the most important aspects and skip over the material you already know well or don't need to know for the exam. Highlighting words, phrases, and facts will help you to see and remember them as you review for your test.

The key to effective highlighting is to be selective. If you highlight every other word or sentence, you defeat your purpose. Too much will be highlighted and nothing will stand out.

So how do you know what's important enough to highlight? Part of it is simply to rely on your judgment. Which facts seem to matter most? Which facts are repeated in the text? Another way you can figure out the important facts in a text is to compare those facts with the information that is tested on the practice tests you find in EMS test-preparation books. If you find that a topic is addressed on several practice tests, you can be sure that the topic warrants highlighting.

You may want to create an intricate system of using different color highlighters for different topics. Or perhaps you want to use one color to highlight key terms and definitions and another color to highlight procedures. Some people find that using too many colors is cumbersome, but others enjoy using a variety of colors.

Benefits of Highlighting

1. It requires you to make decisions about what is important.
2. It focuses your attention on important material.
3. It encourages you to spend more time with that material.
4. It improves your recall of the highlighted material.

Here is an example of how you can use highlighting to draw attention to the important information in a paragraph. Of course, there will be variations in what each person thinks is the most important information, but here's one way to highlight the following passage:

There are three different kinds of burns: first degree, second degree, and third degree. It is important for EMS professionals to be able to recognize each of these types of burns so that they can be sure burn victims are given proper treatment. The least serious burn is the **first-degree burn,** which **causes skin to turn red but does not cause blistering.** A mild sunburn is a good example of a first-degree burn, and, like a mild sunburn, first-degree burns **generally do not require medical treatment** other than a gentle cooling of the burned skin with ice or cold tap water. **Second-degree burns,** on the other hand, do **cause blistering of the skin and should be treated immedi-**

ately. These burns should be **immersed in warm water and then wrapped in a sterile dressing or bandage.** (Do not apply butter or grease to these burns; despite the old wives' tale, butter does *not* help burns heal and actually increases chances of infection.) If second-degree burns cover a large part of the body, then the victim should be taken to the hospital immediately for medical care. **Third-degree burns** are those that **char the skin and turn it black, or burn so deeply that the skin shows white.** These burns usually result from direct contact with flames and have a great chance of becoming infected. **All third-degree burns should receive immediate hospital care.** They should not be immersed in water, and charred clothing should not be removed from the victim. If possible, a sterile dressing or bandage should be applied to burns before the victim is transported to the hospital.

Creating Audio Tapes

To help you learn and review important information, you can use a recording device. Perhaps you want to read aloud unfamiliar information from a textbook into a tape. Or you could simply talk about the new information while the tape player records your observations and connections. The level of formality you use when talking into a tape player is up to you. Some people want to include asides and observations on their audiotapes, while others want to read aloud their texts word for word with no elaboration or extraneous comments. You could experiment with using tapes to remember several of the terms in the glossary of this book. Perhaps you want to read aloud several terms and their definitions onto a tape.

One of the advantages of using audiotapes for studying and reviewing material is that you can listen to the tapes throughout the day while you are driving in your car or going for a jog or waiting in a dentist's office (if you have a Walkman). This way, tapes can help you to space your review throughout the day, which will help to solidify the material in your mind and give you greater flexibility in your study schedule.

If you find that you really like to use audiotapes, you can set up a system of using different tapes for different topics. Then, you can color-code tape labels to keep the categories separate. Or you may want to listen to one tape, and when you feel you know that material, you may want to record new material over it. However you decide to use audiotapes, remember to play back the tapes frequently because repetition is one of the best ways to learn complex information.

Making Connections

Connecting new material that you are learning to something that is already familiar to you will help you to better understand and remember the new material. Think of these connections as individual strings tying each item you want to another and to your brain. When you make several connections among facts or ideas, you have several strings to tie it down in your mind. One string can be easily broken, so the more connections you make, the better. You want to create enough strings to the material to firmly anchor it in your memory.

For example, if you are studying about poisons and want to remember the four ways that poisons enter the body, you could try to make connections to each of the four ways: absorption, injection, inhalation, and ingestion. Perhaps you can recall an incident from your childhood when you or a neighbor accidentally swallowed some poisonous substance (ingestion). Then, scan your mind for a reference to inhalation of a poison and you remember one time when you became dizzy from being in a closed room with a strong household cleaner (inhalation). Do you know of someone who got poison ivy from running in the woods (absorption)? And lastly, think about a friend or a news report about a specific incident involving drugs or a deadly spider (injection).

The key to making strong connections is to create vivid mental pictures of each specific incidence that relates to each term you want to recall. Spend a few minutes thinking about each term so you can create a strong mental image. Go ahead and fill in the details in your mind's eye. Try to involve your other senses as well, by focusing on the smell of a particular poison or how it stung your skin or how foul something poisonous tasted. You'll want to involve as many senses as possible to create truly memorable connections.

You may find that this study strategy works well when you use it to study and recall main ideas, rather than smaller details about a topic. That's because the more detailed the information you want to recall, the less likely you are to know of a specific case you can connect it to in your own experience. In the example above, you can see how creating mental images of past events with which you are familiar could help you to remember the four ways that poisons enter the body. However, to recall more detailed information about poisons, you may want to combine this study strategy with another one. For instance, you could use flash cards to learn how to reduce absorption of a poison across the small intestine (induce vomiting using syrup of ipecac, pump the stomach, or administer activated charcoal).

The last study strategy covered in this book is the use of mnemonics (also known as memory tricks). It is such an important and distinct study strategy that it has its own chapter devoted just to it. See Chapter 3 to learn all about mnemonics.

chapter 3

Mnemonics

Mnemonics are memory tricks that can help you to remember what you need to know. This chapter shows how you can create and use specific mnemonics to help you remember important EMS information for your upcoming exam.

Two popular mnemonic devices, which you may have already used at some time in your previous academic studies, are acronyms and acrostics. Two additional mnemonic devices that are not quite as popular as acronyms and acrostics, but can also be useful, are the place and peg methods. You can also use the technique of visualization to help you recall important information.

The best time to use mnemonics is after you've spent considerable time studying a particular EMS topic. That's because mnemonics help you *recall* information with which you are already familiar—they don't help you to understand *new* material. Now, let's take a closer look at some mnemonics you can use.

CREATING ACRONYMS

The most common type of mnemonic is the *acronym*. An acronym is a word created from the first letters in a series of words. One acronym you may already know is HOMES, which is a word created by using the first letter from each of the names of the Great Lakes:

Huron
Ontario
Michigan
Erie
Superior

You could also make up a silly word to help you remember a list of terms. A common acronym that helps students to remember the colors of the visible spectrum is the nonsense word 'roygbiv.' You could also write the word as a person's name if that helps you to remember the letters: "Roy G. Biv."

Red
Orange
Yellow
Green
Blue
Indigo
Violet

You can create an acronym for just about anything you want to remember. Therefore, you can use acronyms to help you remember the material you are studying for an EMS exam. Even though it will take you a few minutes to create an acronym, that extra time can pay off during exam time when you are able to recall important information. There is no limit to how many acronyms you can create. It's up to you to decide how much time you want to spend creating and memorizing acronyms to help you store and recall the EMS material you need to know on exam day. To begin, just try to create one acronym. See how long it takes you and how comfortable you are with the process. You may then want to try using some of the other mnemonics, too, so you can get a sense of which ones work best for you.

You can follow these seven steps to create your own acronyms:

1. Decide on a particular list of terms you want to memorize or a certain number of steps in an emergency process you want to be able to recall.
2. Write down those terms or steps on a sheet of paper.
3. Take a close look at the letters that begin each word on your paper. Spend a few minutes thinking about those letters.
4. If the order of the terms or steps is not essential, consider the possibility of rearranging the terms.
5. Become creative, and brainstorm to find one or more words that consists of the first letters of the terms in your original list.

6. Pick the acronym from your brainstorming list that you are most likely to remember, based on your own experience, memory, and knowledge.

7. Arrange the terms you want to recall in the order of your chosen acronym. Highlight or make bold the first letter of each term, so that when you review, it will be easier to see the acronym.

Following are two examples of how one student used the seven steps to create an acronym.

Example One

1. I want to memorize the major types of shock.

2. cardiogenic, hemorrhagic, neurogenic, psychogenic, septic, anaphylactic

3. c, h, n, p, s, a

4. The order of terms is not essential: hemorrhagic, cardiogenic, septic, neurogenic, anaphylactic, psychogenic.

5. I could use H. C. SNAP, which stands for a person's first two initials and last name.

6. I can remember H. C. SNAP because I have a friend, Hillary Colleen who likes to snap her fingers when we listen to music, and she likes to shock people by wearing wild outfits.

7. The major causes of shock: H. C. SNAP

> **H**emorrhagic
> **C**ardiogenic
> **S**eptic

Neurogenic
Anaphylactic
Psychogenic

Example Two

1. I want to memorize the signs and symptoms of severe hypothermia.
2. hypotension, undetectable pulse and respiration, stupor or coma, rigidity, eventual ventricular fibrillation
3. H, U, S, R, E
4. The order of terms is not essential: RUSH E; H, U, C, R, E; H CURE; CURE H
5. I could use RUSH E or CURE H.
6. I think I'd be able to memorize RUSH E in relation to hypothermia because when I was a young boy, I was out in a blizzard rushing to my friend's house. I was rushing because I was afraid I would get hypothermia.
7. The signs and symptoms of severe hypothermia: RUSH E

Rigidity
Undetectable pulse and respiration
Stupor or coma
Hypotension
Eventual ventricular fibrillation

Here are two more examples of acronyms that are specifically related to EMS material:

1. To help you remember the basic steps for resuscitation, you can think of the first five letters of the alphabet, ABCDE, which stand for:

> **A**irway
> **B**reathing
> **C**irculation
> **D**rugs
> **E**nvironment

2. To remember the checklist of possible causes for a coma, you can write out the vowels, A, E, I, O, U and then the word "tips":

> **AEIOU TIPS**
> **A**cidosis/alcohol
> **E**pilepsy
> **I**nfection
> **O**verdosed
> **U**remia
>
> **T**rauma to head
> **I**nsulin: too little or too much
> **P**sychosis episode
> **S**troke occurred

Once you invest the time to create several acronyms, review them on a consistent basis. You can rewrite them or read them aloud during your scheduled study sessions. You can also reread them whenever you find a free moment during your day. The key to memorizing mnemonics is repetition, so study your acronyms over and over until they become familiar friends.

CREATING ACROSTICS

Another type of mnemonic is a silly sentence or phrase, known as an *acrostic*, which is made out of words that each begin with the letter or letters that start each item in a series that you want to remember. For example, *Please Excuse My Dear Aunt Sally* is a silly sentence that math students often use to help them remember the order of operations:

> **P**lease **E**xcuse **M**y **D**ear **A**unt **S**ally
> > **P**arentheses
> > **E**xponents
> > **M**ultiply
> > **D**ivide
> > **A**dd
> > **S**ubtract

Here's another example of an acrostic. To recall the letters of the notes on the lines of the treble cleff (E, G, B, D, and F), music students often recite this acrostic:

> **E**very **G**ood **B**oy **D**oes **F**ine

If you know the first letter of a word you cannot recall, your chances of recalling that word are much higher than if you did not know the first letter of it. Therefore, using an acrostic can help you to recall a forgotten word after a few moments of thinking about the letter that word starts with. This can help you to overcome memory block during an EMS exam.

The seven steps for creating acrostics are similar to the seven steps for creating acronyms. The steps are shown on the following page:

1. Decide which terms you want to memorize.
2. Write down those terms on a sheet of paper.
3. Take a close look at the letters that begin each word on your paper. Spend a few minutes thinking about those letters.
4. If the order of the terms is not essential, try rearranging the terms in a few different ways.
5. Spend time brainstorming to create a phrase or silly sentence in which each word begins with the same letter of the terms in your original list.
6. Pick the acrostic that you are most likely to remember based on your own experience, memory, and knowledge.
7. Arrange the terms you want to recall in the order of your chosen acrostic. Highlight the first letter of each term, so that, when you review, it will be easier to recall the acrostic.

Here is an example of how to create an acrostic by using the seven steps above:

1. I want to memorize the signs and symptoms of cardiac compromise.
2. cool and clammy skin, substernal chest pain, abnormal pulse rate or rhythm, radiation of pain to jaw and/or arm, shortness of breath, anxiety, vomiting and nausea
3. C, S, A, R, S, A, V
4. The order of terms is not essential. S, R, S, A, V, C, A

5. Six rosy seals ate very colorful apples. Seven rollicking seals ate very crisp apples.

6. I chose the acrostic "Seven rollicking seals ate very crisp apples" because I like the visual image of seals rollicking; the seven stands for the number of signs and symptoms I need to remember in this acrostic; and when I think of apples, I think of crispness rather than colorfulness.

7. The signs and symptoms of cardiac compromise:

Seven **R**ollicking **S**eals **A**te **V**ery **C**risp **A**pples
Substernal chest pain
Radiation of pain to jaw and/or arm
Shortness of breath
Anxiety
Vomiting or Nausea
Cool and clammy skin
Abnormal pulse rate or rhythm

When creating an acrostic, remember that you'll have an easier time memorizing a phrase or sentence that you can identify with, are interested in, or that you find humorous. So when you get to step six, take the time you need to come up with an interesting phrase or sentence. For instance, if you love to eat sweets, you might want to use words associated with foods when creating an acrostic. Here is an example of an acrostic to help a student remember the order of the superior thyroid artery:

More **I**ce cream **S**hould **S**lowly **C**reate **G**ladness
Muscular
Infrahyoid

Superior laryngeal
Sternomastoid
Cricothyroid
Glandular

Whatever theme you decide to use, don't be afraid to branch out and try others. Creating acrostics is a creative process, so once you get started, you may find it hard to stop!

Here are two additional examples of acrostics:

1. To help you remember the treatment for malignant hypothermia, you could memorize this sentence:

Somebody Help Doug Baker Give
    Icy Fluids Fast, Faster!
Stop triggering agents
Hyperventilate/hundred percent
    oxygen
Dantrolene
Bicarbonate
Glucose and insulin
IV Fluids and cooling blanket
Fluid output monitoring/
    Furosemide/Fast heart
    [tachycardia]

2. To help you remember the list of Ventricular Fibrulation (VF)/Ventricular Tachycardia (VT) drugs used according to Advanced Cardiac Life Support (ACLS), you could use this acrostic:

> **Every Little Boy Must Play**
> **E**pinephrine
> **L**idocaine
> **B**retylium
> **M**agsulfate
> **P**rocainamide

Creating acrostics can help make study sessions fun and interesting. After you create several acrostics, you'll need to review them several times before exam day to make sure they are firmly lodged in your memory. You may want to rewrite them over and over again (using repetition to help you memorize them). Or you may want to read them aloud during your scheduled study sessions. You can also write them on index cards and carry them with you to read whenever you find a free moment during your day. Remember, the best way to memorize mnemonics is through repetition, so spend time reviewing your acrostics until you know them inside out.

ORGANIZING ACRONYMS AND ACROSTICS

Because you will have many terms and definitions to remember for your EMS exam, consider creating a system to help you organize the acronyms and acrostics that you plan to use during your study sessions. A good way to do this is to put the terms you want to memorize into categories by subject. For instance, put together in one group all the terms relating to obstetrics and all those relating to pediatrics in another. This will help you keep track of the mnemonics that you've created during the exam.

You can go a step further in organizing your acronyms and acrostics by using a color-coding system. Use different colored sheets of paper or index cards to create your system. Use a different colored paper or card for each subject. For example, you can write out all the mnemonics you've developed for obstetrics on blue pieces of paper and all those for pediatrics on yellow ones. When you casually glance at your paper, you'll know immediately which mnemonics are related by subject just by noticing the color of the paper the mnemonic is written on.

Keep in mind that each person's subject categories may be somewhat different, and that's okay. One person may put the term *neonate* under the subject of pediatrics and another person may put it under obstetrics. The exact placement of a term in a subject category is not as important as your knowledge of the relationship of that term to other terms in its group. Going through the process of selecting subject categories for your acronyms and acrostics is a good way to get an overview of your EMS study material.

Your list of specific terms to remember in each subject category may differ from another persons because everyone comes to the EMS material with a unique background. Perhaps you already know several of the terms in one subject, but have a hard time recalling any terms in another subject. Some people have nursing experience or other healthcare experience in which they have already learned several medical terms. So each person studying for an EMS exam can focus on the subject categories in which he needs the most practice. The more terms you need to learn, the more acronyms and acrostics you may want to use.

One of the best ways to memorize acronyms and acrostics is through the use of repetition and application to your learning style. If you are a kinesthetic or tactile learner—one who learns by touching or doing—writing out each mnemonic several times will help to seal it in your memory. Auditory learners—those who learn best by listening—might remember the information best if they repeat the acronym or acrostic out loud, over and over. Visual learners—those who learn best by looking—might need to look only at the acronym or acrostic until it is fixed in their minds.

However, you should try to keep several sheets of colored paper or index cards on hand, so you will have an ample supply that will last throughout your entire study plan. You don't want to run out of blue paper just when you come up with a truly terrific acronym or acrostic for those few extra obstetric terms you didn't notice at the beginning of your study schedule. Once you develop a color-coding system, stick to it, so that you don't get confused about which terms go with each color.

One of the benefits of the color-coding system is that even if you forget one of the acronyms or acrostics you create, you may still be able to see in your mind's eye the color of the paper it was written on. On exam day, or in the field, this visualization could help you to recall at least the subject that a term is related to. Believe it or not, you could get an extra point or two just from this knowledge. Here's an example:

In which of these situations should you wear a gown over your uniform?

    a. A 55-year-old man is suspected of having a myocardial infarction.

b. The victim of a fall has no obvious wounds but is
   still unresponsive.
c. A full-term pregnant woman is experiencing
   crowning with contractions.
d. A 72 year-old woman is experiencing dizziness and
   difficulty breathing.

Let's say that after you read the question and all the possible
answers, you are able to narrow the answer choices down to either **a** or **c**. However, you can't remember what "*myocardial infarction*" means. If it has something to do with large amounts of
blood or body fluids, then you would have a difficult time de-
ciding between choice **a** and **c**. A great thing about using a
color-coding system to keep your mnemonics organized into
separate categories is that it can help you recall the subject a
term is related to. So, even though you don't remember the de-
finition of *myocardial infarction*, you do recall that the term was
a part of a mnemonic that was written on purple paper. You
know that all the mnemonics on purple paper are related to the
heart muscle—and the heart muscle is not likely to have a
problem that will expose you to large portions of blood or body
fluids. Therefore, you can confidently pick **c** as the correct answer through the process of elimination.

USING THE PLACE METHOD

One of the oldest mnemonics that is still in use today is called
the method of *loci*; it was first recorded over 2,500 years ago.
Today it is often called the *place method*. The first step in using
the place method is to think about a place you know very well:
perhaps your living room or bedroom. You need to think of a

place that has several items (pieces of furniture or other large items) that always remain in the same place. These items become your landmarks or anchors in the place-method mnemonic. You need to remember where each landmark is in the room and when you visualize walking around this room, you must always walk in the same direction (an easy way to be consistent is to always move around the room in a clockwise direction). Then the next step is to assign an item that you want to memorize to each landmark in your room. A good way to do this is to actually see each word attached to each landmark. Here's an example of how one student uses the place method to remember the structure of the heart. This example uses landmarks in the student's bedroom.

Place Method Example

Landmark		Heart Term
1. Doorway of room	→	1. Aorta
2. Small chair	→	2. Left pulmonary arteries
3. TV stand	→	3. Left pulmonary veins
4. Large vase with flowers	→	4. Left atrium
5. Nightstand	→	5. Left ventricle
6. Bed	→	6. Right ventricle
7. Closet	→	7. Right atrium
8. Bookcase	→	8. Right pulmonary veins
9. Round table with skirt	→	9. Right pulmonary arteries

In this example, the student imagines each part of the heart as being separate from the others and put into or onto each landmark. For example, the aorta is placed in the middle of the doorway to his bedroom. The left pulmonary arteries sit on the small chair, and the left pulmonary veins are shown on the TV that sits on the TV stand, and so on for each item on the list.

To make the place method work, you must first study and understand each term you want to remember, so you can visualize each word and directly link it to each landmark in your chosen place. The more vivid your visualization is, the stronger the connection will be between the terms you want to recall and the landmarks that are already entrenched in your memory.

As you can imagine, it takes some time to create the connections from the landmarks in your special place to the terms you want to remember, but that time will be well spent if it helps you during your EMS exam. The amount of time you spend on creating mnemonics using the place method is up to you; you can spend many hours creating several elaborate place method scenarios, or you can spend a few minutes devising just one.

If you've never heard of the place method before, you may want to start asking waiters and waitresses who don't write down their customer's orders how they remember who gets what. You may find that several waiters and waitresses use the place method to keep track of people's orders because it works so well.

How to USE the Place Method

Understand the information you want to memorize.
Select the landmarks you want to attach the information to.
Encode the landmarks by attaching the information you want to memorize.

USING THE PEG METHOD

The peg method is similar to the place method but it uses numbers and a poem instead of a location as a way to remember important information. An advantage the peg method has over the place method is that you can recall items in any order instead of having to go through the entire sequence to find one of the items in the middle of the list.

The first step in using the peg method is to memorize the simple poem that appears below. You'll need to know this poem by heart, so you can use the numbers in it as the landmarks for linking the new information to. Here is the poem:

> One is a bun
> Two is a shoe
> Three is a tree
> Four is a door
> Five is a hive
> Six is sticks
> Seven is heaven
> Eight is a gate
> Nine is wine
> Ten is a hen

Remember, to make the peg method work, you must commit this poem to memory. Once you memorize the poem, you can use it any time you need to remember things, not just for recalling information for an EMS exam. After you memorize the poem, the next step is to compile a list of terms you want to remember. Then, simply picture the first new term you want to learn with the first word in the poem (bun). Then picture the second word you want to learn with the second word in the poem (shoe). Here's an example of how one student used the peg method to recall the names of the lower extremities.

Peg-Method Example

Word in poem		Lower Extremity Term
1. bun	→	**1.** ilium
2. shoe	→	**2.** acetabulum
3. tree	→	**3.** pubis
4. door	→	**4.** greater trochanter
5. hive	→	**5.** ischium
6. sticks	→	**6.** femur
7. heaven	→	**7.** patella
8. gate	→	**8.** fibula
9. wine	→	**9.** tibia
10. hen	→	**10.** lateral and medial malleolus

In this example, a student ties together in her mind each lower extremity with a word in the poem. The student has already studied a diagram of a lower extremity, so she knows what the terms in the example mean. She imagines the ilium inside of a hamburger bun and the acetabulum sitting inside a shoe. She envisions the pubis in the shape of a tree and the greater trochanter on the front of a door, and so on for each item on the list.

To make the peg method work, you must first study and understand each term you want to remember, so you can visualize each term and directly link it to each word in the poem. The more vivid your visualization is, the stronger the connection will be between the terms you want to recall and the words in the poem that you've already memorized.

USING THE POWER OF VISUALIZATION

Another mnemonic device you can use to help you remember EMS information is the technique of visualization. Visualizing places, people, and scenarios while you are studying can help you to retain important information. While visualization plays an important role in the previous two mnemonics, the place and peg methods, it can also be used by itself without either of those two methods.

Using the power of visualization helps you to be creative when thinking about your study material. Perhaps you like the place method but want to adapt it to fit your own style or needs. Here's one example of how you can use visualization to help you recall important information. In this example, a student visualized specific items in her living room as the landmarks for learning about the heart. She adapted the place method to fit her needs.

Visualization Example

The heart has four chambers.

I am visualizing four items in my living room: gold sofa, brown entertainment center, oriental rug, and grey carpet; these four items are not in the clockwise order that I used for the place method.

The two upper chambers of the heart are called atria (right atrium and left atrium). When I walk in the door to my living room, to the right is a gold sofa (the right atrium), to the left is a brown entertainment center (the left atrium).

The two lower chambers of the heart are called ventricles (right ventricle and left ventricle).

Underneath the gold sofa is an oriental rug (the right ventricle), and underneath the entertainment center is grey carpeting (the left ventricle).

The ventricles are much larger than the atria, just as the rug and carpet are much larger than the sofa and entertainment center.

As you reflect on the example above, you can see how it differs from the place method. The landmarks in the room do not follow a clockwise pattern, and there are only four landmarks as opposed to the nine that were used in the place-method sample. However, you can see how the student adapted the place method by visualizing key terms she wanted to know and linking them to landmarks in her living room. She adapted the place method in this way because she had difficulty remembering which two chambers of the heart are on top and which two are on the bottom. By linking the chambers with her furniture and the carpet and rug underneath that furniture, she was able to quickly remind herself of the correct terms for the upper and lower chambers of the heart.

When you adapt mnemonic devices or create new ones by using the technique of visualization, you interact with your study material in a positive way. That interaction fuels your mind and helps you to get more familiar with the material.

Before you know it, you'll be an EMS expert. Just continue your solid studying habits throughout your EMS career, and you'll be able to pass each new or recertification EMS exam with ease.

chapter 4

EMS Glossary

HOW TO USE THE GLOSSARY

This glossary contains over 650 terms that will be helpful while you are studying for an EMS exam, and after you have passed your exam and are practicing in the field. The terms are listed in alphabetical order. Advanced terms (most likely relevant for EMT-Intermediate or EMT-Paramedics) are designated with an ➤.

A

abandonment   leaving a patient after care has begun and prior to handing care over to someone of equal or greater medical training

abortion   miscarriage; termination of pregnancy, either spontaneously with no known cause or induced

abrasion   a scrape or scratch of the skin

abruptio placenta premature separation of the placenta from the uterine wall. This separation can be partial or complete and is usually painful.

accessory muscles of respiration muscles that aid the diaphragm in breathing, especially when breathing is difficult. These include intercostal muscles, abdominal muscles, and neck muscles.

acclimatization the body's physical adaptation to a different climate or elevation

acquired immune deficiency syndrome (AIDS) the infectious disease that suppresses the body's immune system allowing infections to flourish

activated charcoal a substance that absorbs some toxic ingestions in the stomach and prevents absorption in the body. This is a powder that usually comes premixed with water

acute glaucoma acute rise in eye pressure that can cause permanent blindness if left untreated

acute myocardial infarction (AMI) death of a portion of the heart muscle due to lack of blood and oxygen; a heart attack

adrenergic related to sympathetic nerve fibers of the autonomic nervous system

advanced cardiac life support (ACLS) part of the chain of survival in cardiac care consisting of (1) early access, (2) early CPR, (3) early defibrillation and (4) early advanced care. Advanced cardiac care includes airway control and intravenous drugs.

advanced life support (ALS) the use of invasive or advanced care to sustain life, such as intravenous therapy, medications, endotracheal intubation, etc.

afterload the load against which the left ventricle must pump

agonal usually referring to respirations that are gasping, infrequent, and irregular, typical of a dying patient

airway obstruction blockage of the airway by either a foreign object such as food or by severe swelling of airway tissues

albuterol a bronchodilator medication

➤ **alkalosis** a body pH above 7.45, indicating a low concentration of hydrogen ions

allergen an agent that causes an allergic reaction. Common allergens are insect stings, food, medications, such as penicillin, pollen, and some plants such as poison ivy.

allergic reaction a hypersensitive reaction to an allergen, typically characterized by itching, skin rash, swelling, wheezing, and even hypoperfusion

alveoli the air sacs of the lungs where oxygen and carbon dioxide exchange occurs

➤ **Alzheimer's disease** a type of dementia whereby the patient has progressive loss of mental ability and deterioration of memory

amniotic fluid the fluid that surrounds the baby in the sac prior to birth

➤ **amphetamines** the central nervous system (CNS) stimulant category of drugs that cause general mood elevation, suppress appetite, and prevent sleepiness. This category of drugs is sometimes abused because they can produce euphoria.

anaphylaxis, anaphylactic shock   a severe life-threatening allergic reaction causing hypoperfusion and typically respiratory distress

anemia   low amount of red blood cells in the blood

aneurysm   a ballooning or dilation of a blood vessel (usually an artery) that is weakened for some reason, such as atherosclerosis, hypertension, infection, or trauma

angina   chest pain

angina pectoris   chest pain or discomfort caused by inadequate blood and oxygen to the heart muscle; this condition may be a precursor to AMI

angulated   deformed; at an angle

➤ **antagonist**   a drug that blocks the action of another drug's action

anterior   the front surface of the body or a body part

➤ **anticoagulant**   a drug that inhibits clotting; a "clot buster"

antidote   a substance that will counteract or neutralize a poisonous substance or the poison's effects

➤ **antidysrhythmic**   a category of drugs that manage and prevent ECG rhythm disturbances

➤ **antiemetic**   a category of drugs that reduce or eliminate nausea and vomiting

➤ **antihypertensive**   a category of drugs that manages high blood pressure

➤ **antitussive**   a category of drugs that suppresses the cough reflex

aorta   largest artery in the body. The aorta receives blood from the left ventricle and delivers it to all other arteries.

APGAR   a standardized assessment for newborns taken at one minute and five minutes after birth; the areas of assessment are **A**ppearance, **P**ulse, **G**rimace or irritability, **A**ctivity or muscle tone, and **R**espirations. The scale allows 0 to 2 points for each area making the total score 0 to 10.

apnea   the absence of breathing

arachnoid membrane   the middle of three layers of the meninges; its spiderlike structure gives it this name.

arrhythmia   a disturbance in the heart rhythm or rate

arteriole   a very small artery

arteriosclerosis   an arterial disorder that decreases the arteries' ability to effectively carry blood to the body. The vessels become thickened and lose their elasticity.

artery   a blood vessel that carries oxygenated blood away from the heart

artificial ventilation   breathing for someone by forcing air into the lungs

aspiration   inhaling foreign substance, such as food or vomitus, into the airway or lungs

asthma   a respiratory disorder in which spasm of the small air passages and mucus production occurs, resulting in labored breathing and wheezing

asystole   no electrical impulses in the heart resulting in no pumping and a straight-line ECG reading

atherosclerosis   a thickened, diseased condition of the arteries that prevents the arteries from efficiently carrying blood. The arteries become hardened due to cholesterol build up.

➤ **atrial fibrillation**   an ECG rhythm where the pacemaker is in the atria and electrical activity in the atria is chaotic. This rhythm results in an irregular pulse.

atrium   one of the two upper chambers of the heart (right or left)

➤ **atrophy**   a decrease in cell size due to a decrease in workload

➤ **autoimmunity**   a pathological condition whereby an individual has an immune response to one's own tissues

autoinjector   a type of preloaded medication syringe with a spring loaded action to inject quickly and easily, especially for self-administration such as in a severe allergic reaction

automated external defibrillator (AED)   a portable device that identifies ventricular fibrillation (vf) and either automatically sends a shock or advises that a shock is necessary

➤ **automaticity**   the unique ability of cardiac pacemaker cells to self-depolarize

autonomic nervous system (ANS)   the portion of the nervous system that controls involuntary functions such as cardiac muscle and glands. The sympathetic nervous system and the parasympathetic nervous system are the two divisions.

avulsion   a torn-away or torn-off piece or flap of skin or other soft tissue

B

bag of waters   the sac of amniotic fluid that surrounds the baby in the uterus

bag-valve-mask (BVM) device   a device to provide artificial ventilation to a patient

bandage   a material used to keep a dressing in its place on a wound

➤ **barbiturates**   the category of drugs that depresses the central nervous system. They are used therapeutically to cause sleep and are sometimes abused because they can create a calm, peaceful state.

➤ **baroreceptor**   a sensing mechanism in the aortic arch and carotid sinus that sense any change in pressure in the vascular system

basic life support (BLS)   the use of basic, noninvasive techniques to sustain life or stabilize ill or injured persons

➤ **Beck's triad**   classic characteristics of cardiac tamponade: muffled heart sounds, hypotension, and neck vein distention

➤ **"bends"**   a condition caused by bubbles of gas in the blood that occur during a rapid ascent from deepwater diving

➤ **benzodiazepines**   a category of medications that decreases anxiety and sedate. Diazepam (Valium) and chlordiazepoxide (librium) are common drugs in the category.

beta agonist bronchodilator   a common inhaled medication used for shortness of breath and dilating the bronchi. The medication works by relaxing the muscles surrounding the bronchioles.

beta blocker   a drug that antagonizes actions of the adrenergic receptors of the sympathetic nervous system, resulting in decreased heart rate and dilation of the cardiac vessels

bilateral   both sides

bile   fluid secreted by the liver and stored in the gallbladder to help digest fats

biotransformation   the inactivation of a drug through a metabolic process

bipolar disorder   periods of excessive excitement usually with periods of depression; old term for this is "manic depressive"

blood pressure   the pressure (measured in millimeters of mercury, mmHg) of the blood against the blood vessel wall. The measurement is most commonly taken against an artery.

bloody show   mucous and blood discharge from the vagina; a signal of impending labor

blow-by oxygen delivery   oxygen delivery method for infants by holding the oxygen mask close to the infants mouth and nose but not attaching it

body substance isolation (BSI)   the concept of infection control in which all body fluids or substances are assumed to carry infection

brachial pulse   the pulse point found on the inside of the upper arm; the most common site to check a pulse in infant CPR

bradycardia   a slow heart rate, below 60 beats per minute

brainstem   the lower portion of the brain that is continuous with the spinal cord

breech presentation   the baby's buttocks, legs, arm, or shoulder appear first during birth

bronchi   the two main airway tubes that come off the trachea and go to the lungs

bronchioles   the smaller airway branches that carry air to and from the air sacs

bronchitis   inflammation and irritation of the bronchi, usually chronic in nature. A chronic obstructive pulmonary disease (COPD).

bronchoconstriction   narrowing or constriction of the bronchi

bronchodilator   a medication to open the airways and ease difficulty breathing

➤ **bruit**   a sound emitted when blood meets a partial obstruction. This sound is heard with a stethescope or Doppler.

➤ **buccal**   the inside of the cheek; This is a method of drug administration for some drugs.

C

capillary refill   a simple test to evaluate for hypoperfusion in an infant or child. The examiner presses firmly on the patient's skin to blanch (whiten) the area. In the patient that is perfusing normally, the skin turns pink again in less than two seconds.

With hypoperfusion, the skin may take two seconds or more to pink up.

capillary   the smallest blood vessels where oxygen and carbon dioxide are exchanged

➤ **capnography**   measuring device of exhaled carbon dioxide concentration

carbon dioxide (CO_2)   the gas formed by respiration and exhaled

carbon monoxide (CO)   a poisonous gas created during combustion. It is colorless and odorless.

cardiac arrest   the heart stops beating or pumping

cardiac compromise   a general term referring to a heart related problem

cardiac output   the amount of blood pumped by the heart in one minute. It is calculated by multiplying the stroke volume times the heart rate per minute.

cardiac standstill   cardiac arrest; cessation of the heart

cardiac tamponade   a condition whereby cardiac contraction is greatly reduced due to blood or fluid in the pericardial sac

cardiopulmonary resuscitation (CPR)   basic life support including call for help, initial assessment, opening the airway, artificial breathing, and manual external cardiac compressions

carina   the point in the lower end of the trachea where the two bronchi branch

carotid pulse   the pulse point on each side of the neck; the pulse point checked during adult and child CPR

carotid sinus massage (csm)   use of pressure on the carotid sinus in the carotid artery to convert certain abnormal heart rhythms to a normal sinus rhythm

central nervous system (CNS)   the brain and the spinal cord

cephalic presentation   the normal delivery position where the baby's head appears first during birth

cerebrospinal fluid (CSF)   the fluid that surrounds the brain and spinal cord and their coverings. This fluid is normally clear and watery.

cerebrovascular accident (CVA)   a stroke; lack of blood to a region of the brain, caused by thrombus, embolism, or hemorrhage and resulting in acute symptoms that vary depending on which area of the brain is affected

cervical collar   a rigid brace to stabilize and minimize neck movement after injury or potential injury

chemoreceptor   a nerve cell made active by a chemical stimuli

Cheyne-Stokes respiration   an abnormal breathing pattern sometimes seen with central nervous system problems. The pattern has progressively deepening then shallow respirations with periods of apnea.

cholinergic   effects from the parasympathetic nervous system related to the neurotransmitter acetylcholine

chronic obstructive pulmonary (or lung) disease (COPD or COLD)   a disease of the respiratory system that results in narrowed airways, commonly chronic bronchitis or emphysema, or both

chronic　of long duration

circulatory system　the heart, blood, and blood vessels

clavicle　collar bone

closed fracture　a break in a bone that is not open to the skin

closed head injury　trauma to the head that results in swelling and/or bleeding within the skull

coccyx　tail bone; the lowest bones of the spinal column

cold zone　the noncontaminated safe area at the scene of a hazardous materials incident; this is where the command post and support functions are usually located

colitis　inflammation of the colon

colloid　intravenous solution that contains large molecules such as proteins and starches that cannot pass through capillary membranes

colostomy　the establishment of a surgical opening between the colon and the surface of the abdomen to drain colon contents

coma　a state of total unresponsiveness

comatose　in a coma

concussion　a minor head injury, usually accompanied by transient loss of consciousness

congestive heart failure (CHF)　failure of the heart to effectively pump, causing back up of blood and fluid into the lungs or the body or both. The primary symptom is shortness of breath.

constrict become smaller or narrower

contraindication when NOT to do a specific procedure or give a medication

➤ **cor pulmonale** right-sided heart failure; heart disease that usually occurs secondarily to lung disease

coronary arteries the blood vessels that supply blood to the heart muscle

coronary artery disease the narrowing of the coronary arteries in one or more places. Narrowing can lead to complete blockage, which may cause damage to the heart muscle (AMI).

crackles low pitched, course, abnormal lung sounds caused by fluid in the smaller airways; sometimes called rhonchi

crepitus the grating sound of broken bone ends rubbing together

cricoid cartilage ring-shaped cartilage immediately below the larynx, where an emergency airway may be created

cricothyrotomy an emergency airway established by puncture of the cricothyroid membrane

critical incident stress debriefing (CISD) a group discussion session involving EMS personnel that participated in a particularly emotionally difficult call. The debriefing allows rescuers to discuss the event and their feelings about it.

critical incident stress management (CISM) the collective techniques and methods to assist emergency personnel in coping with very stressful calls, such as line of duty deaths or injuries to children, etc.

croup a common infant and childhood infection characterized by spasm of the larynx or a barking type of cough

crowning when part of the baby's head is seen through the vaginal opening during delivery

➤ **crystalloid** intravenous fluid such as 5 percent dextrose in water (D5W), normal saline, or Ringer's lactate that do not contain protein or other large molecules

➤ **Cushing's triad** signs often observed in a patient with increased intracranial pressure, including a decreased pulse rate, an increase in blood pressure, and change in respirations

cyanosis a bluish or gray color of the mucous membranes and skin, usually around the mouth, fingertips, or earlobes, which indicates severe lack of oxygenation to body tissues

D

➤ **decerebrate** the posture of an unconscious patient in which the arms and legs are extended. This posture usually indicates severe intracranial pressure on the brainstem for some reason.

➤ **decompression sickness** the "bends"; nitrogen trapped in body tissues, having the potential of getting into the blood stream; it is usually related to too quick of an ascent in scuba divers

decontamination the removal of dangerous chemicals or infectious agents

➤ **decorticate** the posture of an unconscious patient in which the arms are flexed and the legs are extended or possibly flexed.

This posture indicates increased intracranial pressure and significant brain injury.

defibrillation electrical shock through a patient's heart to correct ventricular fibrillation

deformity an abnormal shape

dehydration loss of body water

delirium an acute confusional state

▶ **delirium tremons (DTs)** the most severe complication of alcohol withdrawal; symptoms include restlessness, agitation, hallucinations, trembling hands, and possibly seizures. DTs can be life threatening.

delusion a false belief

dementia mental confusion and deterioration over a period of time

dermis the second layer of the skin, found right below the epidermis

diabetes (diabetes mellitus) a deficiency or absence of insulin production by the pancreas, rendering the body unable to use sugar

diabetic coma severe diabetic ketoacidosis; severe hyperglycemia due to inadequate insulin, causing unresponsiveness and possibly death

▶ **diabetic ketoacidosis** hyperglycemia with acidosis and the production of ketones

diaphoresis perspiration

diaphragm　the major muscle of respiration that separates the chest from the abdomen

diastole　ventricular relaxation

diastolic (blood) pressure　the arterial pressure when the heart is relaxed

dilation　to open, enlarge, or expand in diameter

diplopia　double vision

direct pressure　a method of stopping bleeding that involves putting a firm hold on the bleeding site

dislocation　disruption of a joint

disorientation　unable to discern one's name, location, time, or circumstances

distal　an anatomical term describing a position near to the end of an extremity, or further away from the body; opposite of proximal

distended　swollen, stretched

diuretic　"water pill"; a medication used to increase excretion of water from the body; used for treatment of congestive heart failure

diverticula　pockets of weakened areas of the colon wall

diverticulitis　inflammation of diverticula

dorsal　an anatomical term referring to the back or posterior side of the body

dorsalis pedis (pedal pulse)　a pulse in the top of the foot

"downer"　a slang expression for a medication that will depress the central nervous system and cause relaxation and slowing

dressing   protective covering for a wound to help stop bleeding and prevent contamination

drowning   death from submersion (in water)

dura mater   the outermost and strongest layer of the meninges, the covering of the brain

dys   a prefix meaning difficult or painful

dysfunction   abnormal or disturbed function

dysmenorrhea   painful menstruation

dysphagia   difficult or painful swallowing

➤ **dysplasia**   abnormal change in cell, sometimes indicating a precancerous state

dyspnea   difficulty or labored breathing

dysrhythmia   disturbed cardiac rhythm

➤ **dystonic reaction**   muscle stiffness or contractions that may cause distortion and twisted movements, typically in facial or neck muscles, and related to ingestion of some categories of medications

dysuria   painful or difficult urination

E

ecchymosis   bruising

eclampsia   "toxemia of pregnancy"; a severe complication of pregnancy characterized by seizures and preceded by headaches, swelling (edema), and high blood pressure

-ectomy   a suffix meaning surgical removal

ectopic pregnancy　a pregnancy or implanted fertilized egg outside the uterus, most commonly in the fallopian tube and then called a "tubal pregnancy"

edema　swelling of tissues from extra fluid

effacement　the thinning of the cervix in preparation for delivery

efficacy　a drug's ability to produce an expected result

effusion　fluid leakage into a cavity, such as a joint or pleural space

electrocardiogram (ECG)　a graphic representation of the electrical activity of the heart produced by the depolarization and repolarization of the atria and ventricles

electrode　a wire or patch that connects the patient to an electrocardiogram (ECG) machine and measures the electrical activity of the heart

electrolyte　a substance that, when put in water, separates into particles that can conduct an electric current

embolis　blood clot, or fat particle, or air bubble in the blood stream

embolism　movement of a blood clot, fat particle, or air bubble in a blood vessel

emesis　vomit

-emia　a suffix meaning blood

emphysema　a chronic obstructive pulmonary disease (COPD) consisting of the loss of elasticity of the lungs

encephalitis   inflammation of the brain

endocarditis   inflammation of the inside lining of the heart

endocardium   the thin inside lining or membrane of the heart

endocrine system   the body system that produces hormones

endotracheal tube   a tube placed in the trachea to more directly and effectively ventilate a patient and protect the lungs from aspiration

enteritis   inflammation of the small intestine

enzyme   a protein that stimulates and hastens a chemical reaction

epi-   a prefix meaning over or upon

epidermis   the top or outer layer of skin

epidural hematoma   a condition is which blood accumulates in the epidural space

epidural space   the potential space between the dura mater and the skull

epiglottis   the flap of tissue above the larynx (voice box) that closes off the airway when a person swallows

epiglottitis   the inflammation and swelling of the epiglottis, usually by bacterial infection, and potentially life threatening due to airway obstruction

epilepsy   a general term for a seizure disorder that does not have a known cause other than abnormal focus of electrical activity in the brain

epinephrine (adrenaline) a medication administered for anaphylaxis and severe allergic reaction; it opens the bronchi and restores circulation; also, a naturally occurring hormone secreted by the adrenal gland causing the pulse to increase and vasoconstriction.

epistaxis nosebleed

erythrocyte red blood cell

eschar the dry, stiff, necrotic tissue resulting from a full-thickness burn

esophagus the muscular tube that carries swallowed food from the throat to the stomach

etiology cause of a disease or condition

evisceration intestines protruding through an abdominal-wall wound

exacerbation a worsening of a disease or condition

exhalation to breath air out of the lungs

expectorant a medication to loosen up bronchial secretions and facilitate the ability to cough the secretions up

exsanguinate bleed to death

extravasation the leakage of fluids out of blood vessels and into the surrounding tissue

extremities the arms and legs

extrication free from entrapment

exudate pus or serum

F

fainting syncope; transient loss of consciousness due to lack of blood to the brain

fallopian tubes the structures that run from the ovaries to the uterus

febrile feverish

feces bowel movement

femoral pulse the pulse point in the groin

femur thigh bone

fetus unborn child

➤ **Fi0$_2$** oxygen concentration of inspired air

fibrillation chaotic, unorganized electrical activity of the heart, which does not result in mechanical pumping

fibula the smaller, outermost bone in the lower leg

flaccid weak, flabby, lacking muscle tone

➤ **flail chest** condition in which two or more ribs are broken in more than one place, creating an unstable chest wall that ineffectively supports ventilation; Paradoxical or uneven respirations are a classic sign.

flammable capable of being easily ignited

flowmeter a device connected to an oxygen cylinder that measures the amount of oxygen being delivered

fontanelles the soft spots in the skulls of infants; openings in the skull prior to bone fusion

Fowler's position   semisitting

fracture   a break in a bone or solid organ

frontal   pertaining to the forehead

frostbite   a local cold injury where the tissue freezes and is damaged

full-thickness burn   third-degree burn, affecting all layers of skin

fundus (uterine)   the rounded or top part of the uterus

G

gag reflex   a reflex causing one to wretch or make an effort to vomit, when the back of the throat is stimulated or irritated

gall bladder   an organ in the digestive system that stores bile and is located adjacent to the liver

gangrene   tissue death

gastro   a word root meaning "the stomach"

gastrointestinal   related to the stomach and intestines

genitalia   external sex organs

genitourinary system   the organs of reproduction and organs of urine production and elimination

geriatric   pertaining to the elderly, usually over age 65

gestation   the period from conception to birth

Glasgow Coma Scale   a numeric scale reflecting a quick assessment of central nervous system function. The assessment includes eye opening, verbal responsiveness, and motor responsiveness.

glaucoma abnormally high pressure in an eye, leading to pain, redness and vision loss

glottis opening between the vocal cords into the trachea

glucose sugar used by the body and metabolized to create energy

golden hour the ideal time or goal from a traumatic injury to definitive care in the operating room, giving the trauma patient the best possible chance for survival

Good Samaritan laws state laws protecting individuals who stop to render aid at the scene of an accident outside the hospital. These laws provide immunity or minimize liability when acting to the best of one's abilities and to the level of one's training.

grand mal seizure a generalized seizure with periods of intense involuntary muscle contractions and unconsciousness

➤ **gravid** pregnant

➤ **gravidity** the total number of pregnancies including miscarriages

H

hallucination a sensation (visual, auditory, tactile) that does not exist in reality

hallucinogens a group of mind-altering drugs that create hallucinations or distort reality

head-tilt, chin-lift maneuver   a method of opening the airway when the patient is free from a neck or spinal injury

heart attack   a nonmedical term for an acute myocardial infarction; heart-muscle damage due to lack of blood flow

heat cramps   lower-extremity and abdominal-muscle cramping from fluid and salt loss in a hot environment

heat exhaustion   a condition of weakness and dizziness due to excessive fluid loss from heat exposure

heatstroke   sunstroke; severe hyperthermia due to exposure to high environmental temperatures

Heimlich maneuver   a procedure designed to rid the airway of an obstruction of foreign material consisting of a series of thrusts to the abdomen

hem   a root word indicating blood

hemat   a word root meaning "blood"

➤ **hematemesis**   vomiting blood

hematocrit   the percentage of red blood cells in a sample of whole blood; normal value is from 40 to 50 percent, depending on gender

hematoma   a collection of blood in the tissues from an injured blood vessel

hematuria   blood in the urine

hemi-   a prefix meaning "half"

hemiparesis   weakness on one side of the body

hemiplegia   paralysis of the lower half of the body

hemodialysis the filtering or removal of waste products from the blood

hemoglobin the oxygen-carrying pigment of red blood cells

hemolysis the breakdown or destruction of red blood cells

hemophelia a blood clotting disorder that is inherited

hemoptysis coughing up blood

hemorrhage bleeding, either externally, where it can be seen and easily identified, or internally, where it may go unnoticed initially

hemostasis stopping bleeding

hemothorax blood in the pleural space, that is between the lungs and the chest wall

HEPA mask a high-efficiency particulate air filter that prevents microparticles from going through the barrier, worn to prevent transmission of airborne communicable disease

hepat a word root meaning "the liver"

hepatitis inflammation of the liver either by a virus or a toxic chemical

herniation the protrusion of an organ through an opening where it does not belong

hip the joint at the top of the thigh, between the thigh and the pelvis

hives skin disorder, frequently allergic, characterized by redness, swelling, and itching

homeostasis the appropriate balance or stability in the body

hormone   a substance created in one part of the body that stimulates or regulates activity in another part of the body

hot zone   an area in a hazardous-materials incident that is contaminated

huffing   street slang referring to illicit or illegal inhalation of chemicals (paint, glue, etc.) to obtain a "high" or altered level of consciousness

human immunodeficiency virus (HIV)   the virus that causes acquired immune deficiency syndrome

humerous   the bone of the upper arm

humidifier   a device with water, attached to the oxygen delivery system, which provides moisture to the oxygen coming from the cylinder

hyper-   a prefix meaning "too much"

hyperextension   the overextension of a limb

hyperglycemia   high blood sugar

hypersensitivity   allergy

hypertension   high blood pressure

hyperthermia   excessive temperature

hypertrophy   an increase in the size of tissue or an organ due to an increase in the size of the cells, rather than an increase in the number of cells

hyperventilation   increased rate and/or depth of respiration

hypo-   a prefix meaning "too little"

hypoperfusion   a state of inadequate perfusion or blood flow to the body; shock

hypotension   low blood pressure

hypothalamus   the portion of the brain that regulates temperature, sleep, appetite, and other body functions

hypothermia   very low temperature

hypoventilation   inadequate or too low ventilation rate or volume to sustain oxygenation

hypovolemia   state of low or inadequate volume in the circulatory system

hypovolemic shock   hypoperfusion due to inadequate body fluid or blood

hypoxemia   inadequate oxygen in the blood

hypoxia   inadequate oxygen in the blood and delivered to body tissues

I

idiopathic   unknown origin or cause

immobilize   to hold a part firmly in place; to restrict motion

immune system   the body's defense system that fights disease and foreign bodies; comprised of white blood cells, the lymphatic system, antibodies, and body functions

implied consent   the principle of consent that assumes a severely sick or injured unconscious person would want medical intervention if he or she were conscious and able to consent

incident command system (ICS)   a mass casualty management system that coordinates emergency response and operations

incontinence   inability to control elimination of urine or feces

indication   when it is appropriate to use a medication or procedure

infarction   necrosis; tissue death due to lack of blood supply

infection   invasion of the body by pathological microorganism, such as a bacteria or a virus

inferior   anatomical relational term indicating away from the head and toward the feet

informed consent   a permission or agreement to medical treatment and/or transport based upon appropriate information

inhalation   breathing in; drawing air into the lungs

inhaler   a medication spray device that provides an aerosol form of medication into the airway, usually a bronchodilator

innocuous   not harmful

inspiration   breathing in; drawing air into the lungs

insufficiency   inadequacy

insulin   the hormone secreted by the pancreas that allows the body to use sugar

insulin shock   severe hypoglycemia; low blood sugar which may be characterized by abnormal behavior, decreased level of consciousness and seizures; the treatment is sugar

integumentary system   the body system consisting of the covering or the skin, hair, nails, etc.

intercostal   the space between the ribs

intramuscular   into the muscle

▶ **intraosseous**   into the bone; an alternate route for fluids and medications for pediatric patients

intravenous (IV)   into a vein

intubation   insertion of a tube; frequently the placement of an endotracheal tube into the trachea

involuntary consent   permission for treatment or transportation against one's will, usually provided by court or statute

ischemia   lack of blood flow to tissue, usually from severe narrowing of an artery or an obstruction

-itis   a suffix meaning "inflammation"

J

jaundice   a yellowish coloration to the skin or eyes due to excessive bile pigments in the blood; usually a sign of liver disease

jaw-thrust maneuver   a method of opening the airway when it is necessary to avoid moving or extending the neck, such as in cases of trauma

joint   place where two bones come together

▶ **jugular venous distension (JVD)**   bulging of the neck veins

K

▶ **ketoacidosis**   a hyperglycemic condition that may occur in diabetics whereby acids and ketones are produced

kidneys paired organs that filter waste material from blood

kinematics the study of motion and energy

Kussmaul respirations respiratory pattern characteristic of diabetic patients in ketoacidosis, resulting in rapid and deep respirations

L

labor muscular contractions of the uterus intended to expel the fetus

laceration a tearing of cutting wound

lactation milk secretion

laryngectomee a patient who has had surgical removal of all or part of the larynx

laryngectomy the removal of the larynx, usually due to cancer of the larynx

laryngoscope an instrument used to directly visualize the larynx, usually for the purpose of placing an endotracheal tube

laryngospasm severe constriction or narrowing of the larynx, often due to an allergic reaction

larynx the voice box

lateral an anatomical term indicating position away from the middle of the body

lateral recumbent position lying on one's side

lesion a general term used to describe an abnormality

leukemia disease of the blood characterized by excessive white blood cells

leukocyte   white blood cell

liability   legally responsible

ligaments   fibrous connective tissue that joins bones to bones and strengthen joints

limb presentation   situation of childbirth in which the infant's leg or arm is the presenting part during delivery

liver   the large solid organ of the right upper quadrant of the abdomen that detoxifies drugs, secretes bile, produces glucose, vitamins, and other substances and other important functions

living will   a legal document of the terminally ill containing specific instructions to express medical decisions when one becomes incompetent; usually intended to prevent resuscitative efforts or mechanical support

log-rolling   a procedure to move a patient while keeping head and spine aligned

lungs   the organs in the thoracic cavity where the exchange of oxygen and carbon dioxide occurs

lymphatic system   the body system responsible for maintaining the internal fluid system of the body

M

malignant   cancerous or likely to become worse and result in death

mandible   the lower jawbone

mechanism of injury   the cause and method of injury; Consideration includes type, intensity, and direction of force, and body parts affected.

meconium   fetal stool

meconium stain   fecal contamination of amniotic fluid, giving off a green or brownish color and indicating a complication of birth

medial   toward the midline or middle

melena   stool containing blood with a black, tarlike appearance

meninges   three layers of brain and spinal-cord covering; the duramater (outermost), the arachnoid, and pia mater (innermost)

meningitis   inflammation of the meninges

menstruation   the monthly female process of sloughing or shedding the uterine lining

metabolism   the biochemical reactions that take place in the body to provide energy, growth, and other bodily functions

metacarpals   the bones of the hand between the wrist and the fingers

metatarsals   the bones of the foot between the ankle and the toes

midclavicular line   an anatomical landmark consisting of an imaginary line from the middle of the clavical downward on the chest

miosis   excessive pupillary constriction

miscarriage   the spontaneous loss of embryo or fetus prior to the twenty-eighth week of pregnancy; also called a spontaneous abortion

morbidity   degree or severity of illness

mortality   death from a disease or injury

mucous membrane   membranes that line many organs and contain mucous producing glands

mucus   slippery secretion that serves to lubricate and protect various surfaces

multiple casualty incident (MCI)   a disaster or incident where there are multiple victims; sometimes determined when the number of victims exceeds the capabilities of the EMS system

musculoskeletal system   the system of bones, joints, muscles, and related structures that enable the body to move and function

mydriasis   pupillary dilation

myocardial infarction   heart attack; death of a portion of the heart muscle due to an inadequate amount of blood supply

myocardium   the heart muscle

N

narcotic   an addictive category of pain-killer medications that are derived from opium. These drugs are sometimes used illicitly to produce euphoria and relaxation.

nasal cannula   an oxygen delivery device consisting of two prongs that go into the nose

nasogastric tube   a tube that is inserted into the nose while the patient swallows and goes into the stomach to allow drainage, feeding, or to wash out stomach contents

nasopharyngeal airway   a nasal airway; a flexible plastic tube that prevents the tongue from blocking the airway and allows air to flow unobstructed; The tube goes from the nose to the posterior nasopharynx.

nasopharynx   back of the throat and nose

nature of illness   a general description of the medical condition causing the illness requiring EMS response

nausea   the sensation of being sick to the stomach, typically prior to vomiting

near drowning   survival after an event of suffocation in water. Complications can cause death at a later time.

nebulizer   a device that delivers water or liquid medication in the form of a fine spray or mist

necrosis   death of tissue

negligence   failure to act as a reasonably prudent person, resulting in harm

nephritis   inflammation of the kidney

nephro   a word root meaning "the kidney"

nephron   the unit of the kidney that does the actual filtration of blood

nervous system   the brain, spinal cord, and nerves

neuralgia   pain from a nerve

neurogenic shock   hypoperfusion due to nervous system dysfunction resulting in dilation of blood vessels

neuroleptic   a category of drugs affecting the nerves; an antipsychotic drug

nitroglycerine a medication to dilate or open up coronary arteries during episodes of coronary distress

non-rebreather mask an oxygen delivery device that contains a mask with a bag and provides for a high concentration of oxygen delivery

normal saline (ns) a 0.9 percent salt (sodium chloride) solution that is similar to body fluid; It can be administered in an intravenous solution or used as an irrigating solution on a wound.

normal sinus rhythm (NSR) the normal rhythm of the heart where the electrical impulse arises from the sinoatrial node and travels through the heart's normal electrical pathways without interference

nystagmus an involuntary rhythmic jerking of the eyeball; sometimes a sign of toxicity, sometimes congenital

O

occlusion a blockage, usually referring to a blocked blood vessel

ocular related to the eye

off-line medical direction indirect medical direction; physician EMS system oversight that occurs before and after the EMS call

➤ **oliguria** none or minimal urine output

online medical direction direct medical direction that includes voice communication between EMS personnel and a physician during medical care

open fracture   a broken bone in which the wound is open to the skin

➤ **ophthalmoscope**   an instrument used to examine the inside of the eye

➤ **organophosphates**   a category of toxic chemicals that are used as pesticides and cause a toxic emergency when absorbed through the skin

oropharyngeal airway   oral airway; a plastic device to be inserted into the mouth and posterior pharynx in an unresponsive patient without a gag reflex to keep the tongue from occluding the airway

oropharynx   area behind the base of the tongue and back of the mouth

orthopnea   needing to sit up to breathe

orthostatic hypotension   a low blood pressure, usually transient, as one changes from a sitting to a standing position

osteoporosis   decrease in bone density, causing an increased likelihood of a bone break, even without much force

➤ **otoscope**   an instrument used to examine inside of ear and nose

ovary   the female sex organ in which eggs and female hormones are produced

ovulation   process whereby an ovum or egg is released, usually once a month

oxygen   odorless, colorless gas that is essential to life. Normal air contains 21 percent oxygen.

P

pallor very pale skin

palpitation a sensation of heart fluttering or irregularity caused by a dysrhythmia

palsy paralysis

pancreas an organ of the digestive system that secretes insulin and digestive enzymes

pancreatitis inflammation of the pancreas

paralysis loss of the ability to move a body part

paranoia abnormal or unrealistic suspiciousness; exaggerated feelings of persecution

parasympathetic nervous system part of the autonomic nervous system that controls vegetative functions of the body such as digestion

paresis weakness

paresthesia numbness or tingling

paroxysmal occurring suddenly and usually intensely

paroxysmal nocturnal dyspnea sudden onset of severe shortness of breath occurring at night, usually because of fluid collecting in the lungs

partial-thickness burn second-degree burn or one in which the top layer or epidermis is burned and some of the dermis is injured

patent open; not obstructed

pathogen an organism that causes infection

pathological   diseased

pedal   pertaining to the foot

pelvis   the bones of the lower trunk of the body

peptic   pertaining to the stomach

percutaneous   via the skin

perfusion   circulation of blood and oxygen to the body and tissues

peri   a prefix that means around

➤ **pericardial tamponade**   *see* cardiac tamponade

pericarditis   inflammation of the pericardium

pericardium   the membrane around the heart

perineum   area between the anus and the external genitalia

peripheral   anatomical term indicating distance or away from the middle

peristalsis   the muscular contractions of the intestines that move food along during digestion

peritoneal cavity   abdominal cavity

peritoneum   the membrane that surrounds the abdominal cavity

peritonitis   inflammation of the peritoneum

personal protective equipment (PPE)   protection from communicable diseases or hazardous materials with eyewear, gloves, gown, mask, helmet or other protective wear

petit mal seizure   an absence or momentary loss of awareness episode without muscle jerking or other motor dysfunction

pH (potential of hydrogen) a scale representing the relative acidity or alkalinity of a substance. The lower the pH, the more acid and the more hydrogen ions. The higher the pH, the greater the alkalinity, and the fewer hydrogen ions. Normal body pH is 7.35–7.45.

phalanges finger or toe bones

pharmacokinetics the study of the action absorption, distribution, metabolism, and excretion of drugs in the body

pharynx the throat

phlebitis inflammation of a vein

phobia a persistent irrational fear

photophobia sensitivity to light

pia mater the innermost layer of the meninges covering the brain

placenta the afterbirth or organ attached to the uterine wall and connected to the fetus to provide oxygen and food, and exchange waste

placenta previa condition in which the placenta is attached very low in the uterus and potentially over the cervical opening; a normal vaginal delivery is not possible in this case

plasma the fluid component of blood

pleura the two layered lining of the lungs

pleural space the potential space between the pleura that normally contains a small amount of fluid

pleuritis inflammation of the pleura

pneumatic antishock garment (PASG) inflatable trouser-like garment that may be effective in managing shock and stabilizing pelvic fractures. The benefits in shock situations have been controversial.

pneumo a word root meaning "the lungs"

pneumonia infection of the lungs

pneumothorax air in the pleural space

poly- a prefix meaning "excessive"

polydipsia excessive thirst

polyphagia excessive hunger

polyuria excessive urination

position of function the body positions that are natural and relaxed and preserve normal function. For example, the position of function for the hand is the wrist and fingers somewhat flexed.

posterior back side of the body or of an organ

postictal the period of decreased level of consciousness that occurs after a grand mal seizure

➤ **potentiation** an enhanced effect of a drug caused by the simultaneous use of another drug

pre-eclampsia a complication of pregnancy where fluid retention, swelling, and hypertension occur. It can progress to life-threatening ecclampsia with seizures and unresponsiveness.

➤ **preload** the amount of blood returning to the ventricle

pressure dressing bulky bandages secured tightly to provide direct pressure and control bleeding

pressure point   the site of a major artery close to the surface of the body where direct pressure can stop bleeding distal to the site

priapism   sustained penile erection, sometimes due to a spinal cord injury or other medical condition

prolapsed cord   an urgent situation during childbirth when the umbilical cord is protruding from the vagina causing the infant's head to compress the cord against the vaginal wall

proximal   an anatomical term meaning "located toward the center of the body;" opposite of distal

psychosis   major psychological disorder in which the patient is unable to discern what is real from what is not

psychotic   a person with a psychosis

pulmonary   having to do with the lungs

pulmonary artery   the major artery coming from the right ventricle of the heart and carrying nonoxygenated blood to the lungs

pulmonary edema   fluid in the lungs

pulmonary veins   the major veins coming from the lungs and carrying oxygenated blood to the left atrium of the heart

➤ **pulse oximeter**   device to measure the oxygen saturation of blood

R

raccoon eyes   bruises around the eye area without a direct blow to the eyes, usually indicating a fracture in the base of the skull; also caused by broken nose, nasal surgery, or any blow to the face

radial   pertaining to the wrist

radial pulse   the pulse point on the wrist; most often used when taking a pulse rate

radius   the bone of the forearm on the thumbside

rales   lung crackles; abnormal breath sounds

➤ **rapid sequence intubation (RSI)**   orotracheal intubation after temporarily paralyzing a patient with drugs

reasonable force   enough force to restrain or subdue

recovery position   a position to assist in airway maintenance in a breathing but unresponsive patient without trauma. The position is on the patient's side so secretions can drain out of the mouth.

referred pain   pain felt somewhere other than the injured or diseased part of the body

reflex   involuntary reaction to a stimulus

renal   pertaining to the kidney

rescue breathing   artificially breathing for a patient who has stopped breathing

respiration   the exchange of oxygen and carbon dioxide

respiratory arrest   cessation of respirations

respiratory distress   difficulty breathing

retractions   a possible indication of respiratory distress where the skin pulls tight around the ribs, above the clavicles, or in the sternal notch during inspiration

retroperitoneum the area behind the peritoneum; the kidneys are located here

rhonchi lung crackles, abnormal coarse, rattling breath sounds

-rrhage a suffix meaning "excessive flow"

rule of nines a method of estimating the total percentage of burned body surface area, using the principle that the adult human body can be divided into anatomic regions with surface areas that are multiples of 9%.

S

saline salt solution

scapula shoulder blade

scope of practice the specified practices and procedures allowed for a specific healthcare provider usually determined by state statute

sedative a category of medications that depresses the central nervous system causing sedation or sleep

seizure a discharge of electrical activity in the brain, causing some type of neurological dysfunction from a mild period of unresponsiveness to a full-body, uncontrollable contraction of a group of muscles

Sellick's maneuver external pressure on the anterior cricoid cartilage to occlude the esophagus and facilitate endotracheal intubation

sepsis infection

serum   liquid portion of blood remaining after coagulation

shock   discharge of electrical energy as in defibrillation

shock   hypoperfusion; inadequate tissue perfusion

sickle cell anemia   anemia with sickle or crescent shaped red blood cells and destruction of red blood cells

side effect   an undesired effect of a drug

skull   the bony structure of the head

sling   a bandage applied around the neck to support and immobilize the lower arm

sniffing position   placement of the child's head when the head-tilt/chin-lift maneuver; this is the desired position for endotracheal intubation.

spasm   a sudden involuntary contraction of a muscle or constriction of a passageway

sphygmomanometer   a blood pressure cuff; a device to measure blood pressure

spontaneous abortion   miscarriage; delivery of the fetus and placenta prior to the twenty-eighth week of pregnancy

sprain   a ligament injury, either by stretching or a partial tear

standard of care   the minimal level of expected care or performance criteria provided in a particular community

stasis   slowing or sluggishness of the flow of a liquid, usually blood or urine

status asthmaticus   a severe asthma attack that is not stopped by epinephrine or bronchodilator administration

status epilepticus repeated seizures or seizure activity without a period of consciousness

stenosis narrowing

sternum the breast bone

steroid a category of medication

stillborn born dead and unable to be resuscitated

stimulant a category of drugs that stimulates the central nervous system and increases body activity

stoma a permanent opening usually in the abdominal wall, made in surgery

strain a minor muscle injury from overexertion of the muscle

stridor a high pitched sound caused by narrowing of the trachea or larynx

stroke a brain attack or cerebrovascular accident (CVA); damage of a portion of the brain due to lack of blood flow causing a variety of neurological symptoms depending on which part of the brain is damaged

sub- a prefix meaning under

subcutaneous the tissue beneath the skin

subdiaphragmatic below the diaphragm

subdural hematoma accumulation of blood between the pia mater and the arachnoid membrane

sublingual under the tongue

superior a directional anatomy term meaning toward the top or the head

supine　lying on the back, face up

supraclavicular　above the clavical

swathe　a cravat tied around a portion of the body to assist in immobilization

➤ **sympathetic nervous system**　part of the autonomic nervous system that readies the body to react to stressful situations

➤ **sympatholytic**　antiadrenergic; a drug that blocks the action of sympathetic nervous system

➤ **sympathomimetic**　a drug that mimics the action of the sympathetic nervous system

➤ **synchronized cardioversion**　an electrical shock through the heart at a specific time during the cardiac cycle intended to terminate specific dysrhythmias

syncope　temporary loss of consciousness; fainting

systemic　pertaining to the entire body system

systole　the contraction of the heart

systolic (blood) pressure　the arterial pressure when the heart is contracting

T

tachycardia　fast heart beat, usually over 100 beats per minute

tachypnea　rapid respiratory rate

tendon　connective tissue that connects muscle to bone

testes　male sperm producing genitalia located in the scrotum

➤ **tetanus**   a bacterial infection causing muscle spasm of the jaw and clenched teeth (lockjaw)

tetany   muscle twitching or spasm

therapeutic abortion   an induced termination of pregnancy for the health of the mother

therapeutic action   the desired effect of a drug

thoracotomy   surgical opening into the chest

thorax   the chest

threatened abortion   vaginal bleeding indicating the possibility or threat of a spontaneous miscarriage

➤ **thrombolytic**   a category of drugs that breaks down or dissolve thrombi

thrombus   a blood clot

tibia   the shinbone or medial lower leg bone

tidal volume   the volume of inspired or expired air in a single breath

tinnitus   ringing or buzzing noise in the ears, sometimes the result of drug toxicity

tolerance   a diminished effect of a drug, requiring an increase dosage to achieve the same effect

tourniquet   a method of external hemorrhage control, used as the last resort to stop bleeding. It is usually a wide plastic or cloth that is wrapped around an extremity and pulled tightly.

toxemia (of pregnancy)   eclampsia

toxic   poisonous

toxin   poison from plants, animal or bacteria

trachea   the windpipe

tracheostomy   a surgical opening into the neck and trachea

traction splint   fracture stabilization device that exerts force to straighten and align the bone ends, usually for a femur fracture

trade name   brand name or manufacturer's name of a medication

transient ischemia attack (TIA)   a "little stroke" or neurological event whereby the symptoms are temporary, lasting less than 24 hours

transverse lie   an abnormal fetal presentation where the baby is not head down but sideways in the uterus

trauma   injury by an external force, usually a physical injury but it can be psychological

traumatic asphyxia   a severe, life threatening injury to the chest that forces blood from the heart to the upper chest, neck, and face

tremor   an involuntary twitching or fine movement, usually of the hand

Trendelenburg's position   position where patient's feet and legs are elevated higher than the head; used for hypovolemic shock

triage   sorting of patients based on priority

trimester   a period of three months, usually in reference to the three periods or trimesters of pregnancy

trismus   jaw muscle spasm causing clenched teeth

tuberculosis   a chronic contagious infection, usually affecting the lungs

tympanic membrane   the eardrum

U

ulcer   open crater like sore on the skin or mucous membrane

ulna   the larger bone of the forearm on the little-finger side

umbilical cord   the cord containing blood vessels that connect the fetus to the placenta

umbilicus   the navel

unilateral   one sided

universal precautions   infection-control concept that every patient is potentially infection carrying and requires use of gloves, mask, protective eyewear when blood or body secretions are contacted.

uppers   slang for a category of drugs that stimulate the central nervous system

urea   a waste product of the body that contains nitrogen

urinary retention   the inability to urinate

urine   fluid secreted by the kidneys and stored in the urinary bladder

urticaria   hives

uterus   womb; the pear shaped internal female reproductive organ

V

vagina   the birth canal

vascular   pertaining to blood vessels

vaso   a word root meaning "vessel"

vasoconstriction   narrowing of the lumen or diameter of blood vessels

vasodilation   widening of the lumen or diameter of blood vessels

vena cava   the major vein of the body that returns blood to the right side of the heart

venereal disease   a sexually transmitted contagious disease

venipuncture   the puncture or sticking of a vein, usually for the purpose obtaining a blood sample or starting an intravenous infusion

venom   poisonous fluid secreted by some snakes and insects

➤ **venous access device (VAD)**   a surgically implanted device to allow continuous access to circulation

ventilation   the provision of air to the lungs

ventricles   the lower heart chambers; also small cavities in the brain that produce and store cerebral spinal fluid

ventricular fibrillation (vf)   an ECG rhythm characterized by chaotic electrical impulses in the ventricle. This rhythm does not result in pumping and consequently is a cardiac-arrest rhythm requiring immediate defibrillation.

ventricular tachycardia   a life threatening rapid ECG rhythm with an abnormal pacemaker, the ventricle. This rhythm may or may not produce mechanical pumping.

vertebra   the individual bones of the spinal cord

vertebral   pertaining to the spinal column

vertex presentation   the normal position of the fetus during delivery, with the head first

vertigo   dizziness or sensation that the room is spinning

viable   potential to survive or live

visceral   internal tissues and organs

vital signs   pulse and respiratory rate, blood pressure, and temperature

vulva   external female genitalia

W

warm zone   in a hazardous-materials incident, the area of lesser danger but still having the potential of exposure to the hazard. Decontamination takes place here.

wheeze   a high pitched whistling noise indicating narrowed lower airways. In some cases, these may be heard without a stethoscope although ordinarily a stethoscope is necessary to hear them. Asthma, COPD, or an allergic reaction may be the cause.

X

xiphoid process   the cartilage at the lower tip of the sternum

Z

zygoma   cheekbone

APPENDIX   Axial Skeleton

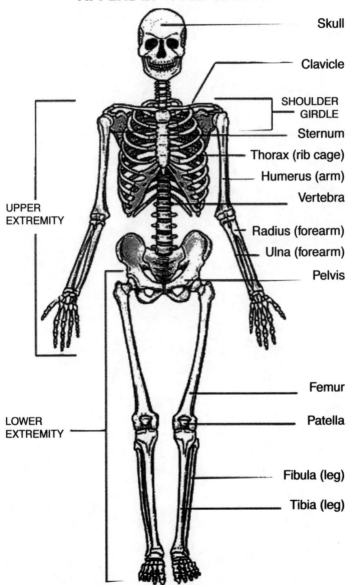

Skull

Clavicle

SHOULDER
GIRDLE

Sternum

Thorax (rib cage)

Humerus (arm)

Vertebra

Radius (forearm)

Ulna (forearm)

Pelvis

UPPER
EXTREMITY

Femur

Patella

LOWER
EXTREMITY

Fibula (leg)

Tibia (leg)

Source: American Academy of Orthopaedic Surgeons (AAOS), *Emergency Care and Transportation of the Sick and Injured*, Seventh Edition, copyright © 1999: Jones and Bartlett Publishers, Sudbury, MA. wwwjbpub.com. Reprinted with permission.